Springer Series on MEDICAL EDUCATION

SERIES EDITOR: Steven Jonas, M.D.

Carole J. Bland, Ph.D., is a Professor in the Department of Family Practice and Community Health at the University of Minnesota Medical School. She directed the federal contract on which much of this text is based. Her research area is faculty and institutional vitality.

Constance C. Schmitz, M.A., is a research fellow with the General College Office of Research and Evaluation at the University of Minnesota. Previously she was a research fellow with the Department of Family Practice and Community Health at the University of Minnesota Medical School. Ms. Schmitz served as project manager and editor for the federal contract in family medicine faculty development on which this text is based. With an M.A. in Curriculum and Instructional Systems and a background in educational publishing, she was naturally interested in the domain of written communication. Currently a doctoral candidate in educational psychology, her professional interests are in program evaluation and outcomes assessment in higher education.

Frank T. Stritter, Ph.D., is a Professor in the Schools of Medicine and Education at the University of North Carolina at Chapel Hill. He was Director of the Office of Research and Development for Education in the Health Professions from 1980 to 1988. His professional interests include curriculum, instruction, clinical education, and faculty development.

Rebecca C. Henry, Ph.D., is an Associate Professor in the Office of Medical Education, Research, and Development of the College of Human Medicine at Michigan State University. Her academic interests include health services research with an emphasis on the physician's role in health promotion and research skill training for health professionals.

John J. Aluise, Ph.D., completed his doctoral studies in organizational development at the University of North Carolina at Chapel Hill in 1982. His professional experience includes marketing research and management training in industry, and faculty appointments in the Business Schools at West Virginia University and Akron University and the Schools of Medicine and Education at the University of North Carolina at Chapel Hill. Dr. Aluise serves as an organizational consultant to academic medical centers and other health care organizations, and his research on the leadership and management of professional organizations has resulted in a major text in the health care field, *The Physician as Manager* (2nd edition, 1988), and numerous chapters and articles.

Successful Faculty in Academic Medicine: Essential Skills and How to Acquire Them

Carole J. Bland, Ph.D.
Constance C. Schmitz, M.A.
Frank T. Stritter, Ph.D.
Rebecca C. Henry, Ph.D.
John J. Aluise, Ph.D.

Springer Publishing Company
New York

Springer Publishing Company, Inc.
536 Broadway
New York, NY 10012

90 91 92 93 94 / 5 4 3 2 1

Library of Congress Cataloging-in-Publication Data

Successful faculty in academic medicine.

(Springer series on medical education ; v. 12)
"Supported in part by funds from U.S.A. Federal Contract # 240-84-0077, Division of Medicine, Health Resources and Services Administration, Department of Health and Human Services."
Includes bibliographical references.
1. Medical education. 2. Medical colleges—Faculty.
3. Medical teaching personnel. I. Bland, Carole J.
II. United States. Health Resources and Services Administration. Division of Medicine. III. Series.
[DNLM: 1. Curriculum. 2. Education, Medical.
3. Faculty, Medical. 4. Professional Competence.
W1 SP685SE v. 12 / W 18 S942]

Library of Congress Cataloging-in-Publication Data
R737.S83 1989   610'.71'1   89-21921
ISBN 0-8261-6730-6

Printed in the United States of America

This book was supported in part by funds from U.S.A. Federal Contract #240-84-0077, Division of Medicine, Health Resources and Services Administration, Department of Health and Human Services.

Contents

List of Tables

List of Figures

Foreword

The year 1989 marks the 10th-year publication for the Springer Series in Medical Education. *Successful Faculty in Academic Medicine: Essential Skills and How to Acquire Them* is the 12th book in the Series. A major focus of our Series has been on teaching and learning in medical school.

Our first book was the ground-breaking *Problem-Based Learning: An Approach to Medical Education* by Howard Barrows and Robyn Tamblyn. We regard student-centered problem-based learning as the wave of the future, as do most current authorities in medical education. We have published two other books on that subject: Dr. Barrows's follow-up book *How to Design a Problem-Based Curriculum for the Preclinical Years* and a description of the pacesetting Primary Care Curriculum at the University of New Mexico, *Implementing Problem-Based Medical Education: Lessons from Successful Innovations*. This work by Dr. Arthur Kaufman and his colleagues concerns the *content* of modern primary care education in medical school as well as the *process* of problem-based learning per se.

Early on we published Robert M. Rippey's *The Evaluation of Teaching in Medical Schools*, still a very useful guide to carrying out that task. More recently, we have turned our attention to faculty development. Calls for major change in both the process and the content of medical education have been made at least as long ago as 1961 (Miller et al.), and more recently by myself (1978), the Association of American Medical Colleges (1984), many of the authors in our Series, and others. Essential, indeed critical, to making positive change in medical education is expansion and redirection of knowledge, skills, and attitudes of medical education faculty, administrators, and staff. The leadership of the change process must also know what to do and possess the skills and attitudes to be able to do it effectively.

To assist in the achievement of this goal, we have recently published three books on faculty development. *Clinical Teaching for Medical Residents: Roles, Techniques, and Programs*, edited by Janine Edwards
and Robert Marier, focuses on a group of *de facto* faculty that with virtually no training in education does a great deal of the clinical teaching of both medical students and junior members of its own ranks. *A
Practical Guide to Clinical Teaching in Medicine*, edited by Kaaren
Douglas, Michael Hosokawa, and Frank Lawler, is aimed at career medical school faculty teaching in the clinical setting.

Now *Successful Faculty in Academic Medicine* presents a grand
design for preparing medical school faculty, admimistration, and staff
at all levels to plan, develop, and implement effective, useful, and educationally sound teaching/learning programs in medical schools. This book
is a guide to curriculum planning, development, and implementation
to achieve this end. Included in the curriculum are the specific types of
the needed knowledge, skills, and attitudes in medical school education,
administration, research, writing, and "professional academic skills."

The audience for this book is variegated: faculty developers—
persons charged with the responsibility for proposing, developing and
implementing fellowships, workshops, and other training experiences
for health care education professionals designed to achieve the goals of
the book; funders of all such medical education reform programs, federal, private, and institutional; the administrators of academic medical
centers who bear the responsibility for making medical education responsive to public need; and last, but certainly not least, the faculty members and fellows in academic medicine who are the means through which
goals of this book will be achieved.

This book "grew out of the special needs to prepare primary care
physicians to succeed as academicians" (p. 7). The recommended curriculum for faculty development focuses on the need for medical educators
to be needs-based and problem-focused in their work, whether it be in
medical student teaching, medical school curriculum design, student
admissions, or student/program evaluation. This book places much practical, "how-to" information on a solid base of research and supporting
documents.

The book stresses the primary importance of establishing and
clearly stating the philosophy of any educational program:

> The building of any curriculum . . . rests on the values and beliefs of
> its architects. How these architects interpret the overall educational
> challenge, how they weigh specific evidence, needs, and arguments, and
> how they choose their methods and materials depends greatly on the
> philosophical perspective they bring to bear. (p. 15)

The authors' own philosophy, based on the work of the educator Ralph Tyler, is neatly summarized in Figure A.1 (p. 279). Goals and competencies are to be specified first, before courses are developed and hours assigned. Achievement of the goals and competencies are to meet specified unmet needs, and they are to do so for one or more reasons, clearly spelled out. The integration of teaching, and learning, and curriculum design is stressed both in the faculty development program itself and in the medical education program that the "developed" faculty and admimistration undertake. Throughout, the close linkage between structure and function, process and content, input and outcome is emphasized.

This book is learner-focused, the learner being the faculty member, the administrator, the medical school staff person. Thus the books approach is the same as the approach that it suggests its users adopt: The focus of their educational work in medical school should be on the learners and their needs, rather than on the faculty and its needs. The volume is "user-friendly," presenting suggestions on "How to Use This Book" (see pp. 10–11). It offers five different plans for achieving its objectives, ranging from a 3-year fellowship to 2-day institutes.

This book is comprehensive in scope, flexible in its potential applications. I hope that it will become a landmark on the road to progressive change in medical education.

STEVEN JONAS, M.D., M.P.H.
Professor
Department of Community and
Preventive Medicine
School of Medicine
State University of New York
at Stony Brook

References

Association of American Medical Colleges. (1984). *Physicians for the twenty-first century: The GPEP report.* Washington, DC.

Jonas, S. (1978). *Medical mystery: The training of doctors in the United States.* New York: W.W. Norton.

Miller, G.E., et al. (1961). *Teaching and learning in medical school.* Cambridge, MA: The Commonwealth Fund/Harvard University Press.

Preface

Although there are over 700,000 full-time academicians in higher education in the United States, and over 60,000 in medical schools alone, suprisingly little has been written about the essential skills required to accomplish the distinct tasks of this profession (Association of American Medical Colleges, personal communication, 1988, Bowen & Shuster, 1986). This book lists those essential skills. It is a significant step, the boldness of which is surpassed only by the detailed plans that follow for teaching faculty members those skills. Together, these skills and suggested learning experiences compose a model curriculum.

We use the term "model" curriculum with some trepidation. There are, of course, many workable plans for any teaching endeavor, innumerable ways to spell out goals and competencies. Some ways are better than others. but can even the most salutary effort, a single gem of a prototype, serve all institutions and all learners? Of course not. As most of you are well aware, contextual constraints, resources, and learner characteristics determine which unique training approach is best for each situation.

Still, there is much to be learned from the articulation and validation of those skills believed to be important for success in an occupational role. The benefit extends not, we hope, to the developers alone, although some research has suggested that curriculum committee members are more deeply affected by curricular reform than either the teachers or students engaged in the "reformed" classrooms! Similarly, there is much to gain from the delineation of courses, activities, teaching strategies, and materials of a potential curriculum—even though they will never be used directly as stated. Such "hypothetical" products show other faculty developers and teachers at least one way to break a path through a rather thick wood; they indicate to funders and sponsors the length and intricacy of the best-laid road; they perhaps inspire the aspiring faculty member with the full challenge of the journey ahead. If one thinks of curriculum development as an instance of problem solving, then the example provided by one carefully worked out solution instructs other encumbered with a similar problem.

This book is about faculty development. It grew out of a federal contract in family medicine faculty development and has now been expanded to focus on faculty development in primary care. It is written primarily for faculty developers, for government and private funders of faculty development, and for the university, college, or hospital administrators responsible for authorizing faculty development activities for their staff. Its content, however, deals with career information that can have enormous value for individual faculty members, particularly prospective and junior faculty. While in tone and language we address the primary audiences mentioned above, we encourage individual faculty members to contemplate the skills and materials presented here.

There is quite a story behind the two-and-one-half-year project that produced this curriculum. Funded by the Division of Medicine, Department of Health and Human Services (DHHS), the contract to "prepare family physicians to perform their faculty roles in university- and community-based educational programs" engaged the full- or part-time work of many professionals from campuses and organizations across the country. For those interested in curriculum development methodology, those simply curious about our activities during those years, or questioning the basis for the skills and courses proposed here, the Appendix provides a summary account of the project. Full documentation of our activities can be found in the *Final Report and Final Curriculum* (Bland et al., 1986). Results of several surveys that were designed to aid the curriculum development process have also been reported in the literature (e.g., Bland, Hitchcock, Anderson, & Stritter, 1987; Bland, Schmitz, Stritter, Aluise, & Henry, 1988; Bland & Stritter, 1988; Hitchcock, Anderson, Stritter, & Bland, 1988; Stritter, Bland, & Youngblood, 1986). For readers whose primary interest is the curriculum itself, Chapter I briefly summarizes the key events of the project that served as cornerstones to the curriculum.

In fashioning this book from the original contract document, we recognized that several components of the curriculum were at least 2 years old. Each of the subject matter domains, therefore, has been updated and revised and a fifth implementation plan has been added. The curriculum was overhauled with the larger primary care audience in mind. What had been the technical report accompanying the curriculum was condensed and moved to the Appendix. We hope these alterations have resulted in a more readable text for audiences more concerned with the curriculum itself rather than our methods of designing it.

This project represents the work of many people who shared an interest in faculty development and who contributed their time and expertise in a variety of ways. We would like to acknowledge their contributions.

First, we are indebted to the Division of Medicine, DHHS, for recognizing the importance of curriculum development in primary care faculty development. In addition to providing financial support for this project, they have been major funders of faculty development in primary care for the past decade.

The authors were actively supported and advised by two committees composed of eight experienced faculty and eight seasoned department chairs who represented a cross-section of M.D.s and Ph.D.s from university- and community based programs in family medicine. (These advisors are listed at the conclusion of this section.) These committees reviewed important drafts of the curriculum and met with us twice for marathon discussions. The authors always came away much enlightened after these meetings.

We would especially like to thank five advisory committee members who also functioned as physician consultants for the authors. Edward J. Shahady, M.D., assisted Dr. Stritter in the Education domain and gave the authors an insightful review of the entire curriculum as well. Robert E. McArtor, M.D., worked closely with Dr. Aluise on Administration. Stephen A. Gehlbach, M.D., M.P.H., assisted Dr. Henry on Research. Robert B. Taylor, M.D., provided Ms. Schmitz with personal materials and an expert reading for the domain of Written Communication. Robert E. Rakel, M.D., gave thoughtful attention to the comparatively new area of Professional Academic Skills developed by Dr. Bland. We are also indebted to the four experts in faculty development and curriculum design who reviewed the first complete draft of the curriculum in early August 1986. Katharine Munning, Ph.D., from Duke University, Stephen Abrahamson, Ph.D., from the University of Southern California School of Medicine, Ilene Harris, Ph.D., from the University of Minnesota, and Robert L. Blake, Jr., M.D., from the University of Missouri/Columbia collectively spent 8 solid days critiquing the curriculum and leading us toward final revisions.

Any project of this size necessarily depends upon the resourcefulness, resiliency, and expertise of its support staff. We were fortunate to have personnel who exceeded expectations on all counts. We wish to thank Pat Youngblood, M.A., at the University of North Carolina for her assistance in preparing requisite competencies and the anno-tated bibliographies in Education and Administration, and in data programming and analysis for the Survey of Selected Exemplary Faculty. Ms. Youngblood filled in many administrative cracks in a timely, professional manner. Also, our thanks to Ms. Karen Boatman, who patiently developed and revised the curriculum maps that describe each of the model approaches to faculty development. Last, but not least, we greatly appreciate the many talents of Jacqueline Hanson and Linda Jagerson at the University of Minnesota, who typed all the documents, coordinated the dissemination of materials, and transferred data and manuscripts.

This book is the result of a core group effort. Together, five content experts worked in surprising harmony with unusual energy and commitment through two and one half years of meetings and suc-cessive curriculum drafts to produce the original reports, and again for 6 months of revision and editing to produce this book. While each content expert should be largely credited with the material presented in his or her domain, the group shares the philosophy and opinions exhibited by the curriculum as a whole. As such, the members of this team are true co-authors.

CAROLE J. BLAND, PH.D.
CONSTANCE C. SCHMITZ, M.A.
FRANK T. STRITTER, PH.D.
REBECCA C. HENRY, PH.D.
JOHN J. ALUISE, PH.D.

Department Advisory Committee

Jack Colwill, M.D., University of Missouri at Columbia

Fitzhugh Mayo, M.D., Medical College of Virginia

Robert E. Rakel, M.D., Baylor College of Medicine

Christian Ramsey, M.D., University of Oklahoma

Edward Shahady, M.D., University of North Carolina at Chapel Hill

H. Thomas Wiegert, M.D., American Embassy, APO, New York

Thomas Nicholas, M.D., University of Missouri at Kansas City

Robert B. Taylor, M.D., Oregon Health Sciences University

Faculty Advisory Committee

William A. Anderson, Ph.D., Michigan State University
Alfred O. Berg, M.D., University of Washington
Stephan A. Gehlbach, M.D., M.P.H., University of Massachusetts at
Amherst
Maurice A. Hitchcock, Ed.D., Family Practice Development Center,
McLennan County Medical Education and Research Foundation,
Waco, Texas
Cynda Johnson, M.D., University of Kansas Medical Center
Robert E. McArtor, M.D., Aultman Hospital, Canton, Ohio
J. Christopher Shank, M.D., Fairview General Hospital, Cleveland,
Ohio
W. Perry Dickinson, M.D., University of South Alabama

References

Bland, C. J., Hitchcock, M. A., Anderson, W. A., & Stritter, F. T. (1987, August).
Faculty development fellowship programs in family medicine. *Journal
of Medical Education, 62*(8), 632–641.
Bland, C. J., Schmitz, C. C., Stritter, F. T., Aluise, J. A., & Henry, R. C. (1988,
June). Project to identify essential faculty skills and develop model cur-
ricula for faculty development programs. *Journal of Medical Education,
63*(6), 467–469.
Bland, C. J, & Stritter, F. T., Schmitz, C., Aluise, J., & Henry, R. C. (1986,
December). *Final report on a model curriculum to prepare family medicine physicians to assume the role of new faculty members in either
university- or community-based educational programs* (HRSA contract
#240-84-0077 Document #HRP 0907077). Springfield, VA: National
Technical Information Service.
Bland, C. J., & Stritter, F. T. (1988, July/August). Characteristics of effective
family medicine faculty development programs. *Family Medicine, 20*(4),
282–288.
Bowen, H. R., & Schuster, J. H. (1986). *American professors: A national
resource imperiled.* New York: Oxford University Press.
Hitchcock, M. A., Anderson, W. A., Stritter, F. T., & Bland, C. J. (1988, Janu-
ary/February). Profiles of family practice faculty development fellowship graduates, 1978–1985. *Family Medicine, 20*(1), 33–38.
Stritter, F. T., Bland, C. J., & Youngblood, P. (1986, March). *Survey of exemplary faculty identified by 50 offices of medical education* (in-house report
for HRSA Contract #240-84-0077). Chapel Hill: The University of North
Carolina, Office of Research and Development for Education in the
Health Professions.

CHAPTER 1

Introduction to the Curriculum: Faculty Members in Academic Medicine and The Need For, Definition, and Uses of a Model Faculty Development Curriculum

It is 3:30 a.m. at the University Medical Center. Associate Professor Dr. Sharon Allen is sitting in the doctor's lounge waiting for Ms. Logan Anderson to reach the final stage of labor. Sharon delivered the Anderson's first two children and has watched them grow through their periodic visits to her family practice clinic. Even after delivering hundreds of babies, Sharon feels that there is something indescribably fulfilling about bringing a newborn baby into the world.

Experience tells her, however, that Ms. Anderson has at least an hour of dilation to go. Anticipating this wait, Sharon brought her briefcase with her and now begins to peruse the enclosed files. Of all the tasks and responsibilities before her, which should earn this time?

One file contains 15 course objectives for a clinical medicine course she directs at the medical school. She and her co-teachers are developing a new exam to assess students at the end of the course. They have decided to try

1

a type of Objective Structured Clinical Exam (OSCE), an approach to assessment that Sharon has read about but never actually used. She and her colleagues are excited about OSCEs because they closely approximate real practice. The challenge, she realizes, lies in constructing valid and reliable performance assessment stations.

A second file contains the computerized statistical printout from her latest research on training primary care physicians to help patients stop smoking. Previous studies suggest that physicians can be very influential in smoking cessation, and smoking is a major health risk among her young, female, indigent patients. The data before her compare patient cessation rates across several physician training programs. Unfortunately, loss of patients from one training group was high; she will have to consult a statistician to learn how to use analysis of variance on groups with unequal numbers.

A third file contains applications from potential students to medical school. The Admissions Committee, which she chairs, has required so much time that last fall she began reading about organizational management and trying various strategies to make the committee more efficient. She enlisted graduate students from the Program in Higher Education Administration of the College of Education to conduct a formal evaluation of her leadership style and the committee's procedures. Committee members now report on the applicants using a standard format; they are responsible for clarifying admissions criteria with the medical school. This week the graduate students will be presenting their final recommendations to the entire committee—that should prove interesting! Who would have ever thought she would be concerned about leadership issues and executive management strategies?

As she ponders which task to tackle she laughs to herself. If she added folders for her residency teaching materials, her student advising lists, grant applications, unpublished manuscripts, clinic schedule, and personal calendar, this briefcase would embody the many roles she plays as an academic professional in primary care. And to quote Jimmy Stewart, "It's a wonderful life!"

The life of a faculty member can indeed be wonderful, or joyous, as Sinderman (1985) concludes in *The Joy of Science*. As one faculty member who participated in a national study of the professoriate said, "there's nothing in the world that will touch it [an academic career]! I hear about all these high rollers and all their [material] things, but they don't interest me at all. They don't know what it is to match wits with people whose wits are worth matching! . . . I *like* the profession. . . " ("Special report," 1985, p. 39).

As the contents of Dr. Allen's briefcase illustrate, however, the life of a faculty member can also be complex, even stressful, given its intellectual demands. The role demands made upon faculty in research, teaching, and service are fairly clear. The junior faculty member is told, "you are to teach, conduct research, and participate in department governance." But what, exactly, does this mean? What skills and abilities are actually entailed?

From a faculty development standpoint, this situation translates readily enough to two central questions. First, what specific nonmedical skills do physician faculty need in order to succeed in academic medicine? Second, how can these skills be intentionally, and efficiently acquired as opposed to haphazardly or idiosyncratically obtained?

This book addresses these questions. It resulted from a two-and-a-half-year effort to study those necessary skills—to identify, describe, and test them—and to propose model plans for teaching them through a faculty development curriculum. Chapters 2 to 9 of this book contain the curriculum itself; Chapter 1 provides a context for it by introducing readers to the problems and issues of faculty development and to the potential use of curriculum components. Let us begin by introducing you to the most important element of all—our "subjects," the faculty members themselves.

Faculty Members in Academic Medicine

Who are the intended learners of this curriculum? They are medical faculty. These people of substantial learning who are employed within (or contribute a significant amount of volunteer time to) a medical school or residency training program. These people typically engage in teaching, research, related public service, institutional service, and patient care. Faculty members are usually appointed (full- or part-time) to one of several tracks: "preceptor" (clinical), "non-tenure-track," and "tenure-track." Expectations for faculty in these various tracks (and even the tracks themselves) vary considerably among institutions. Still, broad generalizations can be made. The following definitions of each faculty role are used throughout this book:

1. *Preceptors* are practicing physicians in the community who work part-time or on a volunteer basis for community- or university-based programs. Their primary task is to supervise students or residents on their clinical rotation.

As such, they are teachers and critical role models for learners: They expand learners' clinical knowledge, demonstrate clinical skills, and evaluate learner performance. Ideally, preceptors should be able to articulate their clinical reasoning process. They should be able to explain how they arrive at certain management decisions and to describe their approach to patients. Consciously or unconsciously, preceptors introduce or expose learners to the values, standards, and daily routine of medical practice.

•   **2.** *Non-tenure-track faculty* have either full- or part-time appointments at university- or community-based programs working both with students and residents. Their primary tasks lie in teaching, patient care, and administration. While they seldom lead a research project, they may be asked to collaborate on a study (by collecting data, for example). As part of their teaching tasks they conduct rounds, precept in the clinic, advise students, and deliver instruction via lecture, small group discussion, and seminar.

        As such, they are, like preceptors, primary role models for learners: They communicate basic knowledge, demonstrate clinical skills, discuss ethical issues, and access the research literature in medicine and education. They provide feedback to learners during instruction and evaluate their learners' performance using several assessment methods.

        Their administrative responsibilities may include setting up, monitoring, and evaluating residencies as well as coordinating clinic operations. In addition, faculty in this role will probably serve the institution (i.e., department, hospital, or university) by sitting on admission, curriculum, and other committees.

        3. *Tenure-track faculty* work full-time in university and sometimes community settings conducting research, in addition to teaching residents and students, providing patient care, and administering projects and programs.

        As such, the teaching and administrative responsibilities listed for non-tenure-track faculty apply here, although the number of hours devoted to teaching may be less. In addition, tenure-track faculty actively develop knowledge in research content areas and conduct research studies. They should promote the discipline and profession by publishing, by participating in national organizations, and by communicating with a network of colleagues. Most likely they will sit on the same committees as non-tenure-track faculty and also those with governance responsibilities, such as judicial committees, faculty senate, and academic freedom and responsibility committees.

        In our research for this curriculum, we discovered that there are some important distinctions between tenure-track faculty in community settings or comprehensive universities and those in research-oriented universities, in terms of their responsibility for and expertise in research. In comprehensive institutions, teaching, service, and research are fairly equally addressed. For this reason, the curriculum identifies four, rather than three, audiences or types of faculty learners: preceptors, non-tenure-track, tenure-track in comprehensive universities or the community, and tenure-track in research universities.

Tenure-track faculty in research-oriented institutions resemble most closely scholars in the basic sciences or other disciplines within higher education. According to Shils (1983, p. 3), these faculty are concerned with "the methodical discovery and teaching of truths about serious and important things... The discovery and transmission of truth is the distinctive task of the academic profession, just as the care of the health of the patient is the distinctive task of the medical profession, and the protection, within the law, of the client's rights and interest is the task of the legal profession."

Bowen and Schuster (1986) argue that academic professionals play a disproportionately important role in society. A surprising assertion? Perhaps so, inasmuch as most faculty conduct their work with little public recognition. "Their work, and its significance, is not widely observed, understood, or appreciated. Faculty members seldom become celebrities" (Bowen & Schuster, 1986, p. 14). Yet through their research faculty advance civilization's technology and recorded knowledge. Through their teaching, they influence the ideas and development of a large percentage of the population. Faculty shape and train essentially all of the professional leaders and most of the business and political leaders in the country. In academic medicine, faculty have a profound effect on the evolving practice of health care in this and other countries.

The academic life in medicine is particularly challenging because of the diversity of roles thrust upon the faculty member and the high performance expectations and accountability built into most of those roles. How do the multiple roles in academic medicine merge within a single faculty member? How do these "process" skills intertwine with the core of medical "content" knowledge that is the physician faculty member's specialized training?

The seasoned faculty member relies on academic skills and uses them daily alongside of his or her medical expertise. Consider, for a moment, "Dr. Stanley Levin," a successful primary care faculty member, who begins the day by attending a medical school senate meeting where discussion concerns changing the curriculum from one based on subject matter domains to one using a problem-based approach. During the debate, Dr. Levin mentally recalls both university and medical school rules and regulations and considers how they might conflict with or impede the principles of problem-based learning. He weighs the advantages of both curricular schemes and estimates the time, costs, and process demands of developing the new curriculum. Education theory, administrative know-how, and a vision of the doctor he wishes to develop are working hand-in-hand.

Later in the morning, Dr. Levin conducts rounds with the general internal medicine residents, simultaneously applying principles of good patient care, modeling those skills for students, briefly lecturing students on related research, and assessing students' physical diagnosis and communication skills. Within each 10-minute visit, Dr. Levin interweaves pedagogical skills (i.e., didactic, small group discussion, student evaluation) with medical knowledge and expertise.

When preparing a research grant proposal that afternoon, Dr. Levin once again draws upon his clinical knowledge. He also accesses his knowledge of the research literature, familiarity with funding agencies and their policies and priorities, understanding of human subjects review guidelines, experience in research design, and skills in technical writing.

Without the ability to explain, demonstrate, listen, assess, and give feedback, the most able physician is ineffectual as a teacher. Without the ability to work in groups, to understand the multiple governance systems in an academic medical center, to organize tasks, and to manage and motivate professionals, the smartest medical specialist is counterproductive as an administrator. Without the ability to critically read and integrate research literature, to design investigations, and to communicate in writing the results of those investigations, the most competent doctor is unable to contribute to knowledge in the area and is limited in his or her career advancement in academe. For these reasons, the "process skills" (what we call the nonclinical skills) of academe are critical for physician faculty.

The Need for Faculty Development Curricula

This book grew out of the special need to prepare primary care physicians to succeed as academicians. These faculty members, like their medical colleagues in general, have been well trained in their physician roles but essentially untrained to succeed as educators, researchers, scholarly writers, or administrators. Our fictional characters, Dr. Allen and Dr. Levin, did not learn academic skills of curriculum development, instruction, evaluation, research, writing, and administration in medical school. Neither did they acquire the necessary value system of academe in medical school. Today's core of primary care faculty have had to learn these skills and values on their own, on the job, sometimes with formal assistance (i.e., faculty development workshops or fellowships), but more often by trial and error or more informal means.

The majority of nonprimary care physician faculty have had some formal training in research through foundation or National Institutes of Health (NIH) programs such as their Institutional Training Grants, New Investigator Research Awards, and Research Career Program Awards. Until recently, however, NIH programs were designed to prepare medical researchers only in specialized "institute areas" that did not include the primary care specialties of general internal medicine, general pediatrics, and family medicine. Thus, faculty members in these disciplines have been especially unprepared for the research tasks awaiting them in university settings.

Like their counterparts in higher education generally, however, many medical schools developed in-service training efforts to prepare and assist faculty in their teaching and administrative rules (e.g., Edwards & Marier, 1988; McGaghie & Frey, 1986, Stritter, 1983). Some of these efforts were greatly augmented by dollars from the federal government, which initiated faculty development training programs for family medicine in 1978. The Kellogg Foundation and the Robert Wood Johnson Foundation, long dominant forces in training clinical scholars, began funding 2-year fellowships to train research-oriented faculty in family medicine. In 1980 the federal government also began funding faculty development programs in general internal medicine and general pediatrics. By 1988 the federal government had supported faculty training for primary care faculty members in over 70 institutions.

The initial focus of these programs was clear: Primary care departments needed faculty, and they needed faculty who could teach. As the years passed, many development programs expanded their goals to include other skill areas such as research, administration, and grant writing, but clinical teaching remained the enduring focus, especially for the federally supported programs in family medicine.

By the early 1980s primary care faculty development found itself at a crossroads; no longer was there consensus on the priority needs of faculty. In addition, there was a dearth of clear models of effective faculty development programs, strategies, and materials. A plethora of "homespun" courses had appeared during the first 10 years, some of which had great merit but others of which lacked in quality. Knowledge of essential faculty skills and successful curricula remained largely unconsolidated. The important lessons concerning effective strategies lay unsummarized. We, and others, felt that faculty development could benefit from "model" programs and courses developed by an experienced, broadly based group of experts.

For this reason, officials in the Division of Medicine (Department of Health and Human Services) decided to fund a two-and-a-half-year curriculum development project. The goals of the contract were to identify important training needs; to research and articulate critical faculty abilities; and to recommend formats, strategies, and materials for training physicians in their faculty roles. Anticipated outcomes of the project included (1) up-to-date information on the requisite faculty skills and (2) useful curriculum materials for designing or revising faculty development programs.

The resulting contract awarded to Carole J. Bland at the University of Minnesota and Frank T. Stritter at the University of North Carolina at Chapel Hill was implemented from June 1984 through December 1986. The resulting materials (Bland, Stritter, Schmitz, Aluise, and Henry, *Final Report and Curriculum*, 1986) provided the stimulus for this book and supported much of the work appearing on the following pages.

Defining "Model Curriculum"

What a "Model" Curriculum Contains and How You Can Use It

A curriculum can be thought of as having two components: *content*, which refers to particular subject matter areas and the attendant knowledge, skills, and attitudes belonging to those areas, and *process*, which refers to an overall structure or scheme for transmitting that content. In this curriculum, the content is divided into five subject matter domains: Education, Administration, Research, Written Communication Skills, and Professional Academic Skills. Each is defined (and defended!) in later chapters of this book.

Curricular process is handled in two ways. First, within each domain, we offer possible course configurations, activities, and teaching strategies as well as suggest current books and other resources for teaching the subject matter. Second, in the chapter entitled "Implementation," we discuss how all five domains may be combined into integrated faculty development programs for different types of faculty at different kinds of institutions. To diagram visually how this integration may be achieved, we have prepared five implementation plans or "maps"; each provides a scheme for sequencing courses within and between the individual domains.

Readers will notice that while the subject matter domains and implementation plans form the heart of the curriculum (if not the bulk of pages), four other components appear in the Table of Contents: Philosophy, Goals and Competencies, Evaluation, and Guidelines for Implementing Faculty Development Programs. As later comments will explain in greater detail, these sections place the content and process of curriculum into a larger context. Philosophy addresses the rationale and assumptions that guided the development of the curriculum; goals and competencies list in tabular form the specific outcomes expected from the curriculum. Evaluation provides a model and set of strategies to use when judging the success of your efforts. The Guidelines list the noncurricular elements of an effective faculty development program, such as the position of the program in the larger organization.

Altogether, we identified 194 faculty competencies organized under 28 goals. We developed 33 courses or other activities in five subject matter domains, supplying 96 annotated references and over 160 additional references and resources. We constructed five implementation plans for acquiring these competencies, ranging in scope from a 3-year fellowship plan (designed for tenure-track faculty in research-oriented universities) to 2-day institutes (for preceptors and non-tenure-track faculty). We outlined evaluation strategies for assessing program effectiveness and learner outcomes. As part of the development process, we constructed three surveys.

Those of you reading this book are most likely either funders, sponsors, directors, or administrators of faculty development programs in primary care. Possibly you might also be a department or committee chair, a fellowship participant, a teacher, or a researcher. These materials lend themselves to a variety of uses, depending on who is reading them. For faculty developers, they outline specific competencies and subject matter, teaching, and evaluation strategies. For funders or researchers, they provide a current synthesis of research and expert opinion on the relevant faculty skills and effective training formats. For the physician faculty member, they articulate an important set of skills. For department chairs or program directors, they may clarify standards for performance, or simply raise questions about current program guidelines or dimensions.

If one approaches curriculum development as an instance of specialized problem solving, then a "model" curriculum is a well-thought-out, sample solution to a problem. The problem addressed is, as we stated in the initial pages, "What faculty skills are essential for success in academic medicine, and how should these skills be learned?" This "model" is not intended to represent a mold from which other replicas are cast, a pattern against which all future programs are cut. Rather, taken as a whole, the curriculum is a heuristic device that others may use in developing curricula, in writing contract or grant proposals, or in embarking on self-directed learning.

More directly, however, discrete elements such as the goals and competencies can be singled out, adopted "wholesale," or modified for certain faculty members. Looking at the curriculum in terms of its smallest elements (i.e., suggested texts, teaching strategies), readers can find useful aids for a variety of instructional purposes.

Listed below are a few specific ways these curriculum components may be used (singly or together):

1. *Use the goals and competencies to develop a survey of department chairs or residency directors and faculty to assess faculty roles and faculty development priorities within your setting.*

Faculty members and department and program leaders need to come to some agreement on faculty roles and professional priorities in order for faculty development to work. One way to generate consensus on the important goals of development is to develop and administer a questionnaire, then follow up the results with group discussion.

2. *Use the competencies in a needs assessment, either as a prelude to designing your own program, or to tailoring one of the implementation plans provided.*

Use the list of competencies to assess your faculty's need for further development. First, transform the competencies into a self-report inventory or objective rating scale to be administered by a trained interviewer. Be aware, however, that self-report yields considerably less valid information.

3. *Use the goals and competencies to develop your own curriculum.*

Some readers may find the set of competencies helpful, the list of goals relevant and important. Still, the suggested courses, materials, and implementation plans may not fit their particular setting very well. These readers may wish to use only the goals and competencies as starting points, for example, to help develop their own courses or research methodology.

4. *Teach one or several of the domains as designed after conducting a needs assessment and tailoring the material as necessary.*

Readers who are interested in only one or two content areas, or who are introducing new courses slowly over a long period of time, may find individual domains more useful than the integrated plans. Individual domain courses can be adopted singly, or in the suggested sequence as shown on the implementation diagrams, after a needs assessment is done.

5. *Adapt one of the five suggested implementation plans after conducting a broad needs assessment, analyzing the department's goals, and discussing the plan with faculty and other key individuals.*

One of the five implementation plans can be adopted after a local needs assessment assures its relevance and feasibility. Advantages and disadvantages of each plan are offered in the chapter on implementation. Before a major plan is adopted, thorough involvement of faculty and administration is needed. Organizational goals and goals of faculty development need to be clarified; faculty roles and skill requirements need to be thought through.

6. *Use the course descriptions and competencies to help select existing courses, workshops, or external programs for your faculty.*

Building new courses, identifying qualified teachers, and preparing for teaching takes a great deal of time. Before implementing new courses, developers should check out locally available courses in areas such as statistics, research design, teaching, and writing.

7. *Use the curriculum to help select external faculty development programs or fellowships.*

Many medical school departments and other programs cannot afford to build their own faculty development program, but can afford to send several faculty members to receive training elsewhere. Fortunately, several excellent national training programs exist. Check with major professional organizations about these opportunities. Use this curriculum's goals, competencies, and subject matter descriptions to make selection of these programs easier, your decisions more informed.

8. *Use the requisite competencies and supporting literature to prepare your next faculty development grant proposal.*

We often speak of research being valuable; we say its values lies in establishing new knowledge, in building better foundations to support future actions. The results of this project are meant to be used in that spirit. They are meant to stabilize the foundations on which faculty development programs are built. We would be pleased to see future programs adopt any part of this curriculum or to cite this source as a reference.

How the Curriculum Was Designed and Developed

The basis for the skills and learning experiences presented here lies in a systematic approach to curriculum development. (See Appendix for a summary of the project's methodology, or write to the federal National Technical Information Services and request a copy of the Final Report and Final Curriculum by Bland, Stritter, Schmitz, Aluise, and Henry, 1986. This approach was originally defined by Ralph Tyler (1950). Tyler's model, or "rationale," is driven by educational objectives as defined by a variety of sources, principally the *learners*, the *society* in which educational activity occurs, and the *disciplines* engaged. Data on these objectives are gathered, then filtered through one's philosophy of learning and teaching. The outcome of such filtering is a set of goals that determine the structure of appropriate learning centers (domains, or subjects), along with their attendant activities and teaching strategies. In Tyler's model, curriculum evaluation is drawn as the final step.

We spent 18 months gathering data from our three sources representing "learners," "society," and the "disciplines." These data helped define and revise the skills (competencies) and goals. Our process began with content experts in five subject matter areas, who were asked to conduct thorough literature reviews of relevant research and practice in their areas and to prepare annotated bibliographies of seminal works in their fields. Out of these extensive searches, 226 competencies (essential faculty skills) were drawn and shared with physician consultants, who closely reviewed them for relevance and importance.

This initial list of faculty skills was then tested in several forms. First, we asked 16 senior department chairs and faculty members serving on the project's advisory panel to rate in a mailed questionnaire, the worth of each skill. Then, the advisory panel and content experts met for a day-long meeting to review the project and discuss the questionnaire results.

At approximately the same time, a concurrent survey of recent graduates from family medicine faculty development fellowship programs was conducted. A condensed version of the same competencies (developed by the content experts and revised by the advisory panel) was used on this survey. Ultimately, several hundred fellowship alumni rated the importance of these skills and reported other perceptions that helped us to shape the curriculum (Bland, Hitchcock, Anderson, & Stritter, 1987).

Two other surveys were designed to test the importance of skills with other relevant audiences. In one survey, the list of competencies was collapsed under more general headings ("goals") and sent to all family practice department heads and residency directors in the nation. Their ratings were useful in understanding the extent to which particular faculty skills change in different institutional settings. In our third and final survey, the full list of competencies was sent to a select group of outstanding faculty members in primary care. These physician "stars" were nominated to participate in the survey by directors of offices of medical education around the country. Tenure-track, non-tenure-track, and preceptor faculty were queried about the importance of the faculty skills for success in their setting (Stritter, Bland, & Youngblood, 1986).

The last method used to gather input data was that of site visits to nationally recognized faculty development centers or programs. All programs served primary care specialties, and all had been "in business" for several years and had established approaches and (in some cases) teaching materials to share. A standard protocol was used during these visits to draw out summary conclusions and recommendations from the various project directors and participants being interviewed (Bland & Stritter, 1988).

All this information—from formal literature review, collaboration with physicians, consensus meetings with respected leaders, surveys, and site visits—fed the subsequent development of actual courses, activities, teaching strategies, and implementation plans. These process elements of the curriculum were prepared by the five content experts, then brought before the advisory groups for feedback and revision. Finally, the complete curriculum was submitted to four external evaluators for formal critique and recommendations. These evaluators (recognized national experts) represented the fields of faculty development, family medicine, evaluation in the health professions, and curriculum development in academic medicine. These recommendations led to the final round of revisions in 1986 and the final products.

The validity for this curriculum, therefore, rests within this process, which used multiple data-gathering tools to ferret out the perspectives of multiple audiences. Wherever it seemed possible, the best judgment and experience of the five content experts was tested and extended ("triangulated") by survey results, group consensus meetings, and external evaluation. Thus, while Dr. Levin and Dr. Allen presented above are fictional, the essential academic skills described in the following pages are not.

References

Bland, C. J., Hitchcock, M. A., Anderson, W. A., & Stritter, F. T. (1987, August). Faculty development fellowship programs in family medicine. *Journal of Medical Education, 62*(8), 632–641.

Bland, C. J., Schmitz, C. C., Stritter, F. T., Aluise, J. A., & Henry, R. C. (1988, June). Project to identify essential faculty skills and develop model curricula for faculty development programs. *Journal of Medical Education, 63*(6), 467–469.

Bland, C. J., & Stritter, F. T. (1988, July/August). Characteristics of effective family medicine faculty development programs. *Family Medicine, 20*(4), 282–288.

Bland, C. J., Stritter, F. T., Schmitz, C. C., Aluise, J. A., & Henry, R. C. (1986, December). *Final report on a model curriculum to prepare family medicine physicians to assume the role of new faculty members in either university- or community-based educational programs* (HRSA Contract #240-84-0077). Springfield, VA: National Technical Information Service.

Bowen, H. R., & Schuster, J. H. (1986). *American professors: A national resource imperiled.* New York: Oxford University Press.

Edwards, J. C., & Marier, R. L. (1988). *Clinical teaching for medical residents: Roles, techniques, and programs.* New York: Springer Publishing Co.

McGaghie, W. C., & Frey, J. J. (Eds.). (1986). *Handbook for the academic physician.* New York: Springer-Verlag.

Shils, E. (1983). *The academic ethic.* Chicago: University of Chicago Press.

Sinderman, C. J. (1985). *The joy of science: Excellence and its rewards.* New York: Plenum.

Special report on the year of the faculty. (1985). *Change Magazine, 17.*

Stritter, F. T. (1983). Faculty evaluation and development. In C. McGuire & R. Foley (Eds.), *Handbook of research and development in health professions education: A guide to policy.* San Francisco: Jossey-Bass.

Stritter, F. T., Bland, C. J., & Youngblood, P. (1986, March). *Survey of exemplary faculty identified by 50 offices of medical education* (in-house report for HRSA Contract #240-84-0077). Chapel Hill, The University of North Carolina, Office of Research and Development for Education in the Health Professions.

Tyler, R. W. (1950). *Basic principles of curriculum and instruction.* Chicago: University of Chicago.

CHAPTER **2**

Philosophy, Goals, Competencies, and Domains of a Model Curriculum

Philosophy

The building of any curriculum, whether for elementary or secondary schools, professional education, or corporate training, rests on the values and beliefs of its architects. How these architects interpret the overall educational challenge, how they weigh specific evidence, needs, and arguments, and how they choose their methods and materials depends greatly on the philosophical perspective they bring to bear.

To Ralph Tyler (1950), these guiding values and beliefs about the purpose and nature of education constituted the curriculum's philosophy of education. The guiding values and beliefs about the process and context of learning constituted the curriculum's philosophy of learning. We provide our views on these topics, as related to primary care faculty development, in the sections below.

Purpose of Faculty Development

The purpose of primary care faculty development is to prepare physicians for their faculty roles. Its goal is to teach them the faculty skills relevant for their institutional setting and faculty position, and to sustain their vitality both now and in the future.

This definition differs in several ways from the traditional pur-

pose of faculty development programs, as stated in the goals of the
early federal grant support program in family medicine. First, it
clarifies our view that skill requirements vary among institutions and
faculty positions and that development programs should attend to
those differences. Therefore, we do not propose a single best model
of primary care faculty development, but a set of flexible curricular
components to guide users in developing programs for specific faculty
types and specific settings. This approach allows for individual tailoring of programs to a range of competencies and alternate implementation plans.

Second, our definition of faculty development states that lifelong
vitality is a goal of faculty development. Skills training is critical,
but alone it is insufficient for developing and maintaining productive faculty. Vitality is also a function of environmental conditions
and personal and institutional "fit," or match (Schuster & Wheeler,
in press). Ideally, faculty development should be integrated with
organizational development to achieve such a fit and to maintain it
over time. While developing prescriptions to do this lies outside the
scope of this volume, it is important that faculty developers realize
the limitations of skills training alone. Maintaining and developing
a vital faculty and institution requires developing the organization
to facilitate faculty and vice versa.

Third, this definition of faculty development implies that a
broader range of faculty skills is more important than those initially
supported by the federal government grant program. We believe that
the discipline needs to meet challenges in research, organizational
development, and other areas as well as faculty recruitment and
improvement of teaching skills.

For example, primary care specialties are currently trying to
build their disciplines through research. This translates quickly into
the need for more emphasis on research, research colleagues and networks, and publishing skills. Programs need to understand the problems of new faculty members and the reasons for continued faculty
shortages, particularly in family medicine. Ways need to be found to
retain talented faculty and enhance their productivity, not just recruit
them. This translates readily into aspects of organizational support
and the socialization (the teaching of academic culture) to new physician faculty members. A final example includes the far-reaching and
rapid changes caused by HMOs, DRGs, and competition within and
among academic medical centers triggered by the rising costs of health
care. This translates to a tremendous need for both personal career
planning and sophisticated administrative skills, such as strategic
planning and creative management.

This broader purpose of faculty development as we have defined it rests well within the established models of faculty development in higher education developed by Bergquist and Phillips (1975) and Gaff (1976). These models include organizational development and personal development, as well as instructional and curriculum development components. Moreover, a major literature review in faculty development from 1965 to 1985 conducted by Bland and Schmitz (1988) revealed a broadening of development issues, particularly during the last decade. The original impetus for development—improving instructional skills of individual faculty members—has been gradually subsumed in most of higher education by the greater survival needs facing educational program. With these changes, "faculty vitality" (or "institutional vitality") has replaced "faculty development" as the preferred construct. This term seems to better reflect the perceptions that today's faculty development problems are of larger scope, have multiple factors, and require systems-level remedies.

Although primary care programs do not currently share all of the problems of higher education (i.e., tenured-in departments), it will soon share many of them (i.e., declining student enrollments, budget cutbacks). For this reason, the broader faculty development models should be seriously considered by future developers. And while the curriculum materials here deal almost exclusively with skills training for individual faculty members, they are influenced by the broader principles and recommendations found in the higher education literature.

Nature of Faculty Development

To be successful, a faculty development program requires commitment from all members. Responsibility for development (change) must be shared; both the individual and the organization (i.e., department or residency program) must consider development worthwhile, must feel ownership in the program, and must feel rewarded for contributing to it. Development that is imposed "from above" or (conversely) initiated at the grass roots level but never sanctioned by the administration is half-successful at best (Bland & Schmitz, 1986).

This means that the goals of faculty development must be congruent with the department's or program's overall mission. The literature contains many reports of fragmented, episodic faculty development activities that yielded little or no impact because the goals and content of development were irrelevant to, or in conflict with, the mission and policies of the parent organization.

By the same token, the effects of faculty development are likely to be fragmented and inconsequential if individual faculty interests are not taken into consideration, or if they are not coordinated with institutional needs and rewards. When institutional rewards and personal values are in conflict, instruction alone will not remedy the problem.

Process of Learning

It takes time to become an effective full-time faculty member, one who is skilled in teaching, administration, research, and publishing. Physicians are well trained in medicine, but few have any training or experience that prepares them for their nonclinical roles. Who has taught them how to conduct research, write educational texts or scholarly articles, develop and implement program-wide curricular plans, negotiate organizational conflicts, or advise students? Refining these skills takes time. It also requires the willingness to study the literature outside of medicine and health; willingness to learn from a variety of professionals (i.e., behavioral scientists, psychologists, editors); and willingness to participate in interdisciplinary teams.

We believe faculty development programs should adopt a "preparatory approach" (Houle, 1980) model of training for their full-time faculty, and consider these participants as novices in need of structured learning and ongoing support from mentors or consultants. If the development program addresses a wide range of skills over considerable time it should result in an advanced degree, indicating the substantive nature of the training. Within this structure there should be flexibility to allow for individual choice. But the curriculum should be rigorous, it should require substantial effort from participants, and it should reflect a careful sequence of skill-building experiences. Part-time and volunteer faculty will require preparation in a smaller set of competencies than full-time faculty, but this training should still be structured and thoughtfully planned.

To illustrate the reasons for a structured approach, Sherman (1983) studied successful National Institutes of Health (NIH) trainees and found that they differed from their less successful colleagues by the amount of time spent in training and amount of emphasis on research skills. Similarly, in family medicine, the longer fellowship programs with emphasis on research produced faculty who publish more than their counterparts from shorter programs (Bland, Hitchcock, Anderson, & Stritter, 1987). Even after formal training, the new faculty member needs attention and supervision. While the seasoned, highly productive researcher needs an environment that permits autonomy, Katz (1978) found that newly trained researchers require close supervision and direction. In fact, during the first year on the job, the "most significant negative correlate" with research productivity is autonomy. Research by Perkoff (1985) also revealed a high level of dissatisfaction among Robert Wood Johnson Foundation-trained graduates in family practice departments. These new faculty found the lack of supervision, seasoned researchers, and role models to be a major problem when combined with considerable role demands (e.g., perform as research director for the department).

The process of becoming a faculty member is one of professional socialization—a most important career event for any professional. When socialization is successful, its effect is one that distinguishes the productive researcher from the nonproductive researcher as seen in a variety of studies (Bland & Schmitz, 1986). To socialize new faculty to an academic career, we believe, structured skill training, protected (or "sequestered") time, and the guidance and support of mentors are critical.

Context for Learning

Unlike college or graduate school education, faculty development programs engage learners who are already in (or are soon destined to be in) a particular work environment. What we know about effective faculty development and the characteristics of productive researchers suggests that it is important that this environment be supportive of the program's goals. Moreover, it needs to support faculty members in participating in development activities and reward them for acquiring and manifesting the skills, knowledge, and behaviors taught in the program.

In some regards, primary care departments and programs are positive contexts for learning faculty skills. They offer participants direct experience and the opportunity to apply concepts in teaching and research directly to faculty responsibilities. They enable participants to maintain their clinical skills, to receive development in the same location in which they live, and to earn an income. They generally provide participants the opportunity to gain a great deal of administrative and other experience quickly.

These benefits are greatly compromised, however, for many of the more difficult skills being learned. Particularly when new faculty have been insufficiently prepared, direct experience may be overwhelming, or unenlightening at best.

The greatest impediment to learning faculty skills in a primary care context comes from the lack of time and competing demands placed on faculty members. Roles are not always clearly defined; as a result, terrific conflicts can occur. New faculty members are not likely to find enough time budgeted for research. They may have to assume management (leadership) positions early in their careers before they are ready to do so. Faculty are often expected to procure their own salaries, either by treating patients or by obtaining grants—which is difficult for any young faculty member to do. Administration, teaching, and patient care are found to be extremely demanding, yet the institution requires evidence of research productivity for tenure and promotion. These disturbing conflicts, which are well described in McGaghie and Frey's *Handbook for the Academic Physician* (1986), suggest that faculty should be highly prepared in preliminary skills before assuming their first full-time position, and certainly before assuming major faculty roles. These demands also underscore the importance of carefully managed faculty entries, of mentors, and of some protected or sequestered learning time.

A second major impediment is that departments and programs lack the resources (primarily human) they need to carry out faculty development, particularly for the full-time, tenure-track candidate. Many programs are small and their staff already overcommitted. Additionally, senior faculty often lack the very skills in research, organizational development and other domains that new faculty are trying to learn.

Because of these constraints, we feel that better use should be made of regional faculty development training sites. Rather than creating as many development programs as there are departments, the limitations of on-site development need to be carefully weighed and considered in light of faculty's needs. Then development programs should capitalize on the strengths of both external and local programs.

Summary

Primary care faculty development programs have accomplished much over the past decade to recruit new faculty members and prepare them as teachers. Their work is not finished, however. Many faculty still lack teaching skills. The discipline faces challenges in research. The academic medical environment faces fiscal and organizational dilemmas. Departments continue to lose faculty and incur significant faculty shortages. The need for faculty skills is strong in all five domains. These skills require time and commitment to learn. They also require structured time, carefully planned and implemented by people with relevant training, and time to commit to development efforts.

Goals and Competencies

What are the specific abilities that enable the primary care faculty member to be productive, satisfied, and successful? While many studies have looked at the life events (e.g., family background, training institution, mentoring relationship) that predict a successful scientist or teacher, few studies have identified the specific competencies required to succeed in academic medicine. (See Chapter 7 for studies that identify important life events.) Thus, a first step in building this curriculum was to identify the major nonclinical responsibilities of a primary care faculty member. Next, we delineated specific abilities required to successfully fulfill these responsibilities. Then we moved on to developing training experiences to arm faculty with the requisite competencies.

The major responsibilities of any one faculty member (or group of faculty members) vary according to their academic appointment, personal goals, and the mission and priorities of their organization. Despite the differences between people, roles, and contexts, we found considerable consensus in our studies on the basic responsibilities and requisite abilities for four types of primary care faculty: preceptors; non-tenure-track faculty; tenure-track faculty in research-oriented, university-based programs; and tenure-track faculty in comprehensive sites or community-based programs. Chapter 1 and the Appendix contain detailed descriptions of each of these types of faculty.

Table 2.1 lists the full range of nonclinical responsibilities expected of primary care faculty members. Preparing faculty to fulfill these responsibilities is the goal of this curriculum. Thus, we refer to these responsibilities as faculty development goals. The appropriateness or relevance of each goal to preceptor, non-tenure-track, and tenure-track faculty in university and community settings is indicated in Table 2.1 by the X's in the column to the right. When the symbol is enclosed in parentheses (X), the goal is optional for this faculty member. The (X) appears under only the non-tenure-track and community-based, tenure-track heading; it signifies that diverse expectations exist for these faculty members.

This is meant to help readers determine relevant faculty development goals for their faculty. We would like to remind you, however, that each faculty group has unique needs. Thus, these goals should be used as a starting point or in conjunction with a local needs assessment to understand the responsibilities and needs of the faculty group to be addressed. As described in Chapter 1, the specification and assignment of goals to faculty type was based on a review of the literature and surveys of: (1) department heads and residency directors;

TABLE 2.1 Faculty Development Goals (or Major Responsibilities) for Four Types of Primary Care Faculty Members

	Precept	Non-tenure-track	Tenure-track[1]	
The purpose of faculty development is to enable faculty to:				
Education			CB	UB
1. Design educational programs (curricula) with appropriate scope, sequence, and focus for intended learners		X	X	X
2. Develop courses, presentations, and course materials using a systematic approach		X	X	X
3. Teach individuals and small groups in clinic and at bedside	X	X	X	X
4. Deliver instruction to small and large groups in classroom settings, using a variety of strategies		X	X	X
5. Assess student performance	X	X	X	X
6. Evaluate program effectiveness both formatively and summatively		X	X	X
Administration				
7. Understand how environmental pressures and (e.g., economic, political, societal, consumer, and organizational) affect academic medical centers		X	X	X
8. Understand the formal structures of and relationships between the organizations they serve (e.g., department, medical school, and university)		X	X	X
9. Participate in and provide leadership for small and large group academic tasks (e.g., plan residency programs, conduct strategic planning, serve on research committees)		X	X	X
10. Manage self, others, money, and time on various projects/programs		X	X	X

[1] CB = community-based; UB = university-based

[2] Parentheses around X indicates this goal may be optional and will depend on the priorities of the setting and role expectations of faculty.

TABLE 2.1 (Continued)

	Precept	Non-tenure-track	Tenure-track[1]	
			CB	UB
Research				
11. Access and critically read the research literature in medicine, education, and other domains	X	X	X	X
12. Understand theory and empirical findings in one's own research area		(X)[2]	(X)	X
13. Formulate a research question and operationalize variables		(X)	(X)	X
14. Design descriptive and/or explanatory studies		(X)	(X)	X
15. Collect and analyze data		(X)	(X)	X
16. Evaluate and discuss study findings		(X)	(X)	X
17. Conduct and manage research projects		(X)	(X)	X
Written Communication				
18. Communicate effectively to different audiences		(X)	X	X
19. Develop process strategies for organizing and drafting written material		(X)	X	X
20. Prepare material according to general and specific format guidelines		(X)	X	X
21. Apply rules of English usage, style, and composition		(X)	X	X
Professional Academic Skills				
22. Understand the underlying values, traditions, and unwritten behavior codes of academia		(X)	X	X
23. Effectively manage a productive career in academia		(X)	X	X
24. Establish and maintain a network of professional colleagues in academia		(X)	X	X

[1] CB = community-based; UB = university-based

[2] Parentheses around X indicates this goal may be optional and will depend on the priorities of the setting and role expectations of faculty.

(2) exemplary faculty in family medicine and other clinical specialties; and (3) alumni of family medicine faculty development fellowships. (See Chapter 1 and the Appendix for descriptions of the surveys and how the goals for each faculty type were identified.)

Tables 2.2, 2.3, and 2.4 list the specific competencies required to successfully fulfill each of the 24 major nonclinical responsibilities of each faculty type listed in Table 2.1. These 194 requisite competencies were identified by the same methods used to identify the faculty goals. The same goals and competencies are also presented in the chapters on each domain, by content area. If you are interested in seeing all of the goals and competencies related to research, for example, you will find them listed in the chapter on "Research Domain."

In summary, this chapter lists the requisite competencies of the successful primary care faculty member. As such, it serves as the foundation for the rest of the book, which describes how to build programs to help faculty acquire these abilities. The following chapters (3–7) address competencies for the five domains (Education, Administration, Research, Written Communication, and Professional Academic Skills). After these domains are presented, Chapter 8 (Implementation Models) describes five different plans for combining the courses and other learning strategies from all five domains. Each of these models is designed to meet the training goals for one of the faculty types.

One caveat should be given here, and this caveat is repeated throughout the book. The most effective faculty development program will both arm individual faculty members with the requisite competencies listed here *and* create an environment where faculty can use these abilities to their fullest. Without question, there are some essential competencies a faculty member needs to have in order to succeed, but possessing these competencies does not ensure success. In fact, multiple studies conclude that the best predictors of faculty productivity and morale are organizational characteristics such as a critical mass of productive faculty colleagues, appreciative administration, sufficient support resources, and so on (e.g., Bland & Schmitz, 1986; Blackburn, 1979; Corcoran & Clark, 1984).

The Domains

We turn now from the philosophy and goals of faculty development to the specific content to be learned and the courses, activities, and resources for that learning. We have clustered the requisite competencies into five domains: education, administration, research, written communica-

tion, and professional academic skills. The following chapters address each of these domains separately. The chapters begin with an introduction that defines the domain, explains its importance to primary care, and states the authors' assumptions. Then the requisite goals and competencies for that domain (presented earlier in Table 2.4) are listed again. This time a brief explanation accompanies each goal to flesh out exactly what is meant by these short phrases.

Next, suggested courses, strategies, and resources for teaching each competency and achieving the goals of that domain are given. A rationale is then given for why the specific courses are designed as presented and, if appropriate, why a particular sequence of courses is recommended.

Finally, each chapter ends with an annotated bibliography of the 20 or so most relevant references and a complete list of all references cited in the domain.

TABLE 2.2 Faculty Development Goals and Nonclinical Competencies for Tenure-Track Faculty Members

---

Education

GOAL 1.0: Design educational programs (curricula) with appropriate scope, sequence, and focus for intended learners

1.1 Articulate a program purpose
1.2 Identify salient characteristics of potential participants
1.3 Research and synthesize literature relevant to program topics
1.4 Evaluate instructional resources and constraints by analyzing the environment
1.5 Select and sequence curricular content
1.6 Write program goals

GOAL 2.0: Develop courses, presentations, and course materials using a systematic approach

2.1 Translate broad educational goals into specific instructional objectives
2.2 Classify objectives according to types of learning required (i.e., verbal skills, intellectual skills, problem-solving skills, motor skills, and attitudes)
2.3 Develop instructional units from objectives
2.4 Choose a teaching format (e.g., course, readings, preceptorship) appropriate for the instructional purpose
2.5 Apply general principles of adult learning (e.g., set expectations, practice opportunities, evaluate performance, provide feedback)

(continued)

TABLE 2.2 (Continued)

Education

2.6   Plan individual sessions including teaching strategies to be used (e.g., lecture, small group)
2.7   Select or prepare instructional resources and materials such as syllabi, visuals

GOAL 3.0: Teach individuals and small groups in clinic and at bedside

3.1   Clearly explain course objectives and directions to learners
3.2   Help learners organize their learning activities
3.3   Ask questions at various taxonomic levels to stimulate thinking
3.4   Respond to learners so that their interest and involvement in the learning process are strengthened
3.5   Direct learners to the literature and other resources when they lack prerequisite knowledge or have special interests
3.6   Assign outside readings or tasks to reinforce learning
3.7   Describe differences between inpatient and outpatient teaching
3.8   Orient learners to each particular patient care setting
3.9   Help learners set realistic learning expectations by assigning responsibilities appropriate to the developmental stage of each learner
3.10 Insert oneself into the clinical situation to model appropriate practices, attitudes, and interpersonal skills

GOAL 4.0: Deliver instruction to small and large groups in classroom settings, using a variety of strategies

4.1   Research a topic and gather materials for a lecture
4.2   Prepare a written outline for a lecture
4.3   Deliver a lecture that includes the use of audiovisuals, follow-up questions, and discussion
4.4   Coordinate various types of small group instruction (e.g., seminars, simulations, and discussions)
4.5   Develop tasks and/or problems to be addressed by a group
4.6   Lead a discussion and delegate tasks to group members
4.7   Develop simulations to be used by a group

GOAL 5.0: Assess student performance

5.1   Identify different purposes for evaluating performance such as diagnosing learning, assigning grades, and certifying learners
5.2   Use checklists and rating scales when observing live or recorded learner performance
5.3   Keep anecdotal records to evaluate learner progress

TABLE 2.2 (Continued)

5.4 Give learner positive and negative feedback on progress toward achieving course/program objectives

5.5 Counsel learners to help them develop self-evaluation skills

5.6 Understand various mechanisms for evaluating learner progress and choose a method appropriate for a given purpose

5.7 Utilize simulations including print, computer, patients, and videotapes

5.8 Design and conduct oral examinations

5.9 Conduct and interpret simple checks on reliability and validity of evaluation methods

5.10 Design written tests that include objective short answer and essay-type questions

GOAL 6.0: Evaluate program effectiveness both formatively and summatively

6.1 Identify questions, the answers to which will inform specific decisions about the instructional program

6.2 Develop an evaluation plan to include data collection instrument(s) (e.g., questionnaire, interview, test)

6.3 Determine the most appropriate data source(s) (e.g., self, learners, peers, administrators, and/or experts) and collect the data

6.4 Analyze the data and interpret the results

6.5 Report results to concerned individuals

6.6 Revise instruction as appropriate

Administration

GOAL 7.0: Understand how environmental pressures and trends (e.g., economic, political, societal, consumer, and organizational) affect academic medical centers

7.1 Identify the constituencies, such as governmental agencies, industry groups, and large segments of the consumer population, that their organization(s) serve

7.2 Analyze the current economic and political situation(s), research and education trends directly affecting their institution and program

7.3 Contribute to organizational planning and problem solving as it applies to economic and political issues

GOAL 8.0: Understand the formal structures of and relationships between the organizations they (e.g., department, medical school, university) serve

8.1 Determine how their department or program goals relate to the overall mission of the institution

8.2 Describe the parallel faculty and administrative governance structure of their institution

(continued)

TABLE 2.2 (Continued)

Administration

8.3   Describe the institutional and departmental judicial process according to Delbecq's three criteria for justice: representative, structure, visibility of decisions, and clarity of decision-making rules and policies

8.4   Describe the organization's decision-making process regarding finance, personnel, and program responsibilities

8.5   Identify the organization's stage of development: creation, direction, delegation, consolidation

8.6   Evaluate the mechanisms that enhance an organization's strength, such as automation, performance appraisal, management expertise, planning, and evaluation process

8.7   Determine if their organization is receptive to organizational change, and facilitate an appropriate change strategy as an internal change agent

GOAL 9.0: Participate in and provide leadership for small and large group academic tasks (e.g., plan residency programs, conduct strategic planning, serve on research committees)

9.1   Identify personal leadership style
9.2   Use a contingency model of leadership
9.3   Demonstrate group leadership skills to achieve both the task and socioemotional requirements for effective group work
9.4   Identify sources of conflict and apply appropriate strategies to resolve conflict
9.5   Foster a collaborative environment, characterized by respect for differences, freedom of expression, and consensus decision making

GOAL 10.0: Manage self, others, money, and time on various projects and programs

10.1 Establish a self-management system that includes negotiated goals and objectives, multiple evaluation sources, and a regular review and reporting process
10.2 Hire, train, supervise, and evaluate personnel
10.3 Manage their time by prioritizing objectives, scheduling major activities, assigning and delegating tasks, and monitoring work of others
10.4 Conduct effective meetings
10.5 Interpret and prepare financial and other accountability reports

Research

GOAL 11.0: Access and critically read the research literature in medicine, education, and other domains

11.1 Use appropriate resources (libraries, computers) to complete literature searches

TABLE 2.2 (Continued)

11.2 Critically evaluate a research article

GOAL 12.0: Understand theory and empirical findings in one's research area*

12.1 Identify an area of interest in a given body of literature
12.2 Identify experts in that area of interest
12.3 Explain (in a general way) the importance of theory to research
12.4 Relate specific questions of interest to underlying theory
12.5 Pursue an area of interest over an extended period of time, remaining current in pertinent literature
12.6 Recognize the classic studies, traditional designs, common forms of measurement, common variables, and common methodological problems related to one's own research content
12.7 Critically synthesize the literature relevant to one's own research question
12.8 Identify conferences and professional organizations that focus on one's own research area

GOAL 13.0: Formulate a research question and operationalize variables*

13.1 Identify a problem or general question to investigate
13.2 Refine the problem so it can be investigated
13.3 Establish a clear purpose to the research
13.4 Translate the general question into specific hypotheses, recognizing the difference between research, null, and alternative hypotheses
13.5 Define variables and terms operationally
13.6 Recognize the difference between independent and dependent variables when applicable
13.7 Determine how each variable will be measured, recognizing different levels of measurement
13.8 Evaluate the reliability and validity of a given measurement
13.9 Evaluate variables and their measurement in one's area of research

GOAL 14.0: Design descriptive and/or explanatory studies*

14.1 Categorize research designs (e.g., observational vs. interventional, and prospective vs. retrospective)
14.2 State the purpose, strengths, and limitations of each design
14.3 Compare major types of studies, such as case reports, case controls, cross-sectional, longitudinal, and epidemiological studies, clinical trials, survey studies, field research, and evaluation studies
14.4 Explain important threats to internal and external validity applicable in each design
14.5 State the relationship between the chosen research design, the type of data collected, and the necessary statistical techniques

(continued)

TABLE 2.2 (Continued)

Research

14.6   Prepare for and use consultation from design specialists
14.7   Thoroughly analyze the dominant research designs used in one's special area of study
14.8   Recognize sources of error in one's study and methods to minimize error when possible

GOAL 15.0: Collect and analyze data*

15.1   Distinguish inferential from descriptive statistics
15.2   Determine the universe, population, appropriate sample, sample size, and appropriate sampling technique for a given study
15.3   Understand basic statistical concepts such as statistical significance, mean, median, mode, standard deviation, standard error, prevalence rate, incidence rate, and p-value
15.4   Understand commonly used statistical tests such as chi-square, t-test, analysis of variance, correlations, and multiple regression
15.5   Construct a plan for managing data files and for analyzing those data according to their level of measurement and the research design
15.6   Be familiar with available statistical packages (e.g., SPSS, SAS, BMD) to direct computer personnel in what analysis to use and related decisions (e.g., how to handle missing data)
15.7   Interpret printouts on common analyses from available statistical packages (listed above) for one's research area
15.8   Understand how to graphically summarize data (e.g., histogram, bar graph, pie chart, frequency curve)
15.9   Report results correctly and be able to cite strengths and limitations of the study based on the data
15.10 Prepare for and use consultation from computer analysts and statisticians
15.11 Understand more advanced statistical tests used in one's research area, such as discriminant analysis, principal components analysis, and multiple logistic analysis

GOAL 16.0: Evaluate and discuss study findings*

16.1   Explain the outcome of given analyses in terms of the originally stated hypothesis
16.2   Conduct additional literature review as needed to elaborate upon findings and their implications for a given body of research
16.3   Integrate the research findings into the existing literature by discussing what is known, unknown, and what requires further study
16.4   Express appropriate cautions in interpreting results and base these cautions on methodological and theoretical conditions

TABLE 2.2 (Continued)

16.5 Place one's study in the context of existing research and justify how it contributes to important questions in the area

GOAL 17.0: Conduct and manage research projects*

17.1 Develop plans for implementing a study, including timeline, budget and requirements for personnel, facilities, and supplies
17.2 Identify appropriate funding sources (local, state, national)
17.3 Identify faculty collaborators from within and outside the discipline who can offer guidance to the project
17.4 Hire, manage, and evaluate personnel involved with a study
17.5 Prepare and submit required reports, budget requests, and other administrative documents
17.6 Secure permission from human subjects, research, and other institutional review committees and boards
17.7 Implement and direct a research project
17.8 Prepare a research proposal suitable for submission in one's research area

Written Communication

GOAL 18.0: Communicate effectively to different audiences

18.1 Test own methods for knowing one's audience
18.2 Describe both a typical member of the audience and the variety of people that represent it
18.3 Specify the elements of knowledge and experience the audience has (or does not have) related to the topic
18.4 Determine why the audience may want or need one's information or viewpoints
18.5 List the criteria by which the audience will judge one's written material

GOAL 19.0: Develop process strategies for organizing and drafting written material

19.1 State the primary purpose for writing
19.2 Explain what is new, different, or important about the message or content
19.3 List (or diagram) the primary points of the message and their connections
19.4 Determine what background information (facts, definitions, references) readers need in order to understand the content
19.5 Determine boundaries for the subject: which points or topics get included, which excluded
19.6 Establish who's "talking" (writing), in which tense (past, present, future)

(continued)

TABLE 2.2 (Continued)

Written Communication

19.7   Read with a critical ear to develop or test ideas
19.8   Implement a system for abstracting/documenting literature and
       other sources of information on the topic
19.9   Develop whatever intrinsic structure the content has and adapt
       it to the publication format
19.10 Use frameworks for structuring material, such as diagrams and
       notes, content outlines, minidrafts, etc.
19.11 Schedule a timetable for writing that encourages systematic and
       frequent writing sessions
19.12 Build in a mechanism for evaluation and revision (e.g., pilot test,
       second or third readers, editor/proofreader)

GOAL 20.0: Prepare material according to general and specific format
            guidelines

20.1   Summarize the content requirements each format imposes, e.g.,
       (IMRD) introduction, methods, results, discussion, or components
       of a proposal, parts of a book, elements of a student syllabus,
       format for business correspondence, etc.
20.2   Access reference materials that detail stylistic and technical
       conventions of each format (maximum length, reference style,
       headings, tables and graphs, photos, other guidelines for
       preparing manuscripts)
20.3   Decide when and how to deviate from conventional formats
20.4   Determine how the material will be printed, bound, and delivered
       before writing
20.5   Select an appropriate journal for the article
20.6   Follow protocols for submitting and revising manuscripts

GOAL 21.0: Apply rules of English usage, style, and composition

21.1   Avoid faulty constructions such as nonparallel sentence structure,
       dangling participles, misplaced modifiers, run-on sentences,
       disagreement between subject and verb, and conflicting tenses
21.2   Spell correctly
21.3   Punctuate consistently
21.4   Use words precisely, according to their meaning
21.5   List references according to American Psychological Association
       or Index Medicus style
21.6   Access resource and reference material for questions on usage
21.7   Write in the active voice
21.8   Choose definite, specific, concrete words
21.9   Avoid sex-biased or culture-biased language

TABLE 2.2 (Continued)

21.10 Decode jargon for the audience

21.11 Eliminate redundancy

21.12 Avoid pompous and overly tentative statements (two sides of the same coin)

21.13 Vary the pattern of sentence structure; vary adjectives, verbs, and nouns

21.14 Allow humor, warmth, or other expressions of feeling to surface when appropriate

21.15 Edit for economy

21.16 Vary personal style to suit the readers' general background, needs, time frame, and organizational status

21.17 Make all parts of the text relevant to the central purpose and main ideas

21.18 Work within the given structure of the format and the personal outline

21.19 Provide introductory sentences or paragraphs at the beginning of new and summary sections

21.20 Provide transitions when merging ideas, themes, or facts

21.21 Sequence arguments, concepts, and facts in a logical and persuasive manner

21.22 Provide illustrations (verbal or visual), examples, anecdotes, or definitions to suit the audience

21.23 Construct graphs, charts, tables, and figures according to reference guidelines, and base the text on the data as it appears in the visual (not the other way around)

21.24 Proofread for accuracy and completion of design. For example, check that:
  — each chapter is listed on the contents page
  — each reference has a number or citation, and vice versa
  — the abstract covers truly principal features of the study
  — each "patient question" is answered
  — each goal specified has objectives
  — each objective specified has instructions
  — each enclosure promised has been attached

Professional Academic Skills

GOAL 22.0: Understand the underlying values, traditions, and unwritten behavior codes of academia

22.21 Describe what attracts successful academics to the profession (e.g., opportunities to teach, produce new knowledge, determine own area of investigation, enjoy prestige associated with being university professor, contribute to society by ensuring an educated populace)

(continued)

TABLE 2.2 (Continued)

Professional Academic Skills

22.2   Discuss values of academicians (e.g., academic freedom, importance of knowledge production, publishing, patient care, student growth and development)

22.3   Describe how these values do or do not permeate policy and mission of the institution (e.g., Regent's Mission Statement, promotion and tenure code, grievance process, dean's priorities for the school, and priorities of university)

22.4   Identify unwritten rules and practices of academics (e.g., authorship on articles, establishing collaborative research relationships, soliciting information from potential funding sources)

22.5   Discuss values of practicing physicians (e.g., patient care, family, community health)

22.6   Ascertain how well one's own values match with academic and institutional values

22.7   Identify (and adapt to, when appropriate) different value systems within the department, university, practicing community, National Institutes of Health, etc.

GOAL 23.0:   Effectively manage a productive career in academia

23.1   Describe the purpose of one's own superordinate structures (e.g., college, hospital, university)

23.2   Explain the role of one's own unit within the larger organization's goals and purposes

23.3   Describe the administrative structure of the unit and entire organization, naming key people (e.g., department head, dean, vice president, president, board of regents, affirmative action officer)

23.4   Describe faculty authority, governance, and participation within the administrative structure, naming key people (e.g., medical school faculty senate chair, university senate representatives from medical school, senate president, senate committees)

23.5   Describe one's roles, assignments, and responsibilities in the department, college, hospital, and university

23.6   Describe other faculty members' and support staffs' roles in these settings

23.7   Describe daily activities of successful academics (e.g., plan and teach courses; read broadly in areas affecting discipline and institutions; conduct research; participate in local, institution-wide, and national committees and review panels; work in multiple sites—office, clinic, hospital, on the road)

23.8   Identify how faculty activities are influenced by the explicit and implicit expectations of each level of the organization (Levels might include unit, department, college, hospital, and university. Expectations might include "publish 3 articles a year in refereed

TABLE 2.2 (Continued)

journals," "acquire funding for 50% of salary within 2 years through research grants or patient-generated dollars," "teach at all levels of medical education," "participate in university governance through senate membership or promotion review")

23.9 Describe rewards of being productive in the organization (e.g., seeing one's work used, local recognition, public recognition, contribution to knowledge development, contribution to student development, contribution to patient care, opportunities to participate in higher level of governance and administration, promotion, tenure)

23.10 Identify personal goals, interests, and rewards

23.11 Assess how well the organization's goals and expectations match with one's desired activities, goals, and interests

23.12 Identify the required or rewarded products (e.g., publications, grants, awards, promotion packet, patient-generated dollars)

23.13 Identify the maximum time allowed (if one exists) for acquiring rewards (e.g., must be promoted in 7 years or terminated; must acquire grant support in 3 years or salary reduced)

23.14 Identify which level(s) of the organization controls the rewards one values (for example, the department head may expect and reward time devoted to patient care, the university may expect and reward published articles in refereed journals.)

23.15 Identify skills, contacts, and experience one needs to produce valued products

23.16 Develop a promotion packet

23.17 Negotiate assignments, leaves, and responsibilities

23.18 Describe the mission and structure and name the key people of major funding sources, professional organizations, and academic organizations

23.19 Describe purpose and publishing policies of relevant publications

GOAL 24.0: Establish and maintain a network of professional colleagues in academia

24.1 Maintain productive (vs. social) professional relationships with an advisor or mentor(s) and with training peers

24.2 Maintain frequent, substantive contact with productive researchers in one's research area, both within one's institution and elsewhere

24.3 Seek opportunities to collaborate (e.g., combine resources, personnel, activities, goals) across one's network

24.5 Participate in professional groups and activities associated with the college, hospital, university, discipline, research area, or funding sources

*Indicates that these goals and related competencies may be optional for community-based, tenure-track faculty—see Table 2.1.

TABLE 2.3 Faculty Development Goals and Nonclinical
Competencies for Non-Tenure-Track Faculty*

Education

GOAL 1.0: Design educational programs (curricula) with appropriate scope, sequence, and focus for intended learners

    1.1 Articulate a program purpose
    1.2 Identify salient characteristics of potential participants
    1.3 Research and synthesize literature relevant to program topics
    1.4 Evaluate instructional resources and constraints by analyzing the environment
    1.5 Select and sequence curricular content
    1.6 Write program goals

GOAL 2.0: Develop courses, presentations, and course materials using a systematic approach

    2.1 Translate broad educational goals into specific instructional objectives
    2.2 Classify objectives according to types of learning required (i.e., verbal skills, intellectual skills, problem-solving skills, motor skills, and attitudes)
    2.3 Develop instructional units from objectives
    2.4 Choose a teaching format (e.g., course, readings, preceptorship) appropriate for the instructional purpose
    2.5 Apply general principles of adult learning (e.g., set expectations, practice opportunities, evaluate performance, provide feedback)
    2.6 Plan individual sessions including teaching strategies to be used (e.g., lecture, small group)
    2.7 Select or prepare instructional resources and materials such as syllabi, visuals

GOAL 3.0: Teach individuals and small groups in clinic and at bedside

    3.1 Clearly explain course objectives and directions to learners
    3.2 Help learners organize their learning activities
    3.3 Ask questions at various taxonomic levels to stimulate thinking
    3.4 Respond to learners so that their interest and involvement in the learning process are strengthened
    3.5 Direct learners to the literature and other resources when they lack prerequisite knowledge or have special interests
    3.6 Assign outside readings or tasks to reinforce learning
    3.7 Describe differences between inpatient and outpatient teaching
    3.8 Orient learners to each particular patient care setting

TABLE 2.3 (Continued)

3.9 Help learners set realistic learning expectations by assigning responsibilities appropriate to the developmental stage of each learner

3.10 Insert oneself into the clinical situations to model appropriate practices, attitudes, and interpersonal skills

GOAL 4.0: Deliver instruction to small and large groups in classroom settings using a variety of strategies

4.1 Research a topic and gather materials for a lecture
4.2 Prepare a written outline for a lecture
4.3 Deliver a lecture that includes the use of audiovisuals, follow-up questions, and discussion
4.4 Coordinate various types of small group instruction (e.g., seminars, simulations, and discussions)
4.5 Develop tasks and/or problems to be addressed by a group
4.6 Lead a discussion and delegate tasks to group members
4.7 Develop simulations to be used by a group

GOAL 5.0: Assess student performance

5.1 Identify different purposes for evaluating performance such as diagnosing learning, assigning grades, and certifying learners
5.2 Use checklists and rating scales when observing live or recorded learner performance
5.3 Keep anecdotal records to evaluate learner progress
5.4 Give learner positive and negative feedback on progress toward achieving course/program objectives
5.5 Counsel learners to help them develop self-evaluation skills
5.6 Understand various mechanisms for evaluating learner progress and choose a method appropriate for a given purpose
5.7 Use simulations including print, computer, patients, and videotape
5.8 Design and conduct oral examinations
5.9 Conduct and interpret simple checks on reliability and validity of evaluation methods
5.10 Design written tests that include objective short answer and essay-type questions

GOAL 6.0: Evaluate program effectiveness both formatively and summatively

6.1 Identify questions, the answers to which will inform specific decisions about the instructional program
6.2 Develop an evaluation plan to include data collection instrument(s) (e.g., questionnaire, interview, test)

(continued)

TABLE 2.3 (Continued)

Education

6.3 Determine the most appropriate data source(s) (e.g., self, learners, peers, administrators, and/or experts) and collect the data
6.4 Analyze the data and interpret the results
6.5 Report results to concerned individuals
6.6 Revise instruction as appropriate

Administration

GOAL 7.0: Understand how environmental pressures and trends (e.g., economic, political, societal, consumer, and organizational) affect academic medical centers

    7.1 Identify the constituencies, such as governmental agencies, industry groups, and large segments of the consumer population, that their organization(s) serve
    7.2 Analyze the current economic and political situation(s), research and education trends directly affecting their institution and program
    7.3 Contribute to organizational planning and problem solving as it applies to economic and political issues

GOAL 8.0: Understand the formal structures and relationships of the organizations they (e.g., department, medical school, university) serve

    8.1 Determine how their department or program goals relate to the overall mission of the institution
    8.2 Describe the parallel faculty and administrative governance structure of their institution
    8.3 Describe the institutional and departmental judicial process according to Delbecq's terms of three criteria for justice: representative structure, visibility of decisions, and clarity of decision-making rules and policies
    8.4 Describe the organization's decision-making process regarding finance, personnel, and program responsibilities
    8.5 Identify the organization's stage of development: creation, direction, delegation, consolidation
    8.6 Evaluate the mechanisms that enhance an organization's strength, such as automation, performance appraisal, management expertise, planning, and evaluation process
    8.7 Determine if their organization is receptive to organizational change, and facilitate the appropriate change strategy as an internal change agent

TABLE 2.3 (Continued)

GOAL 9.0: Participate in and provide leadership for small and large group academic tasks (e.g., plan residency programs, conduct strategic planning, serve on research committees)

9.1 Identify personal leadership styles
9.2 Use a contingency model of leadership
9.3 Demonstrate group leadership skills to achieve both the task and socioemotional requirements for effective group work
9.4 Identify sources of conflict and apply appropriate strategies to resolve conflict
9.5 Foster a collaborative environment, characterized by respect for differences, freedom of expression, and consensus decision making

GOAL 10.0: Manage self, others, money, and time on various projects and programs

10.1 Establish a self-management system that includes negotiated goals and objectives, multiple evaluation sources, and a regular review and reporting process
10.2 Hire, train, supervise, and evaluate personnel
10.3 Manage their time by prioritizing objectives, scheduling major activities, assigning and delegating tasks, and monitoring work of others
10.4 Conduct effective meetings
10.5 Interpret and prepare financial and other accountability reports

Research

GOAL 11.0: Access and critically read the research literature in medicine, education, and other domains

11.1 Use appropriate resources (librarians, computers) to complete literature searches
11.2 Evaluate a research article critically

---

* The minimum number of goals and competencies for this faculty member have been listed, not the maximum possible [see (X)s, Table 2.1].

TABLE 2.4 Faculty Development Goals and Nonclinical
Competencies for Preceptors

Education

GOAL 3.0: Teach individuals and small groups in clinic and at bedside

  3.1 Clearly explain course objectives and directions to learners
  3.2 Help learners organize their learning activities
  3.3 Ask questions at various taxonomic levels to stimulate thinking
  3.4 Respond to learners so that their interest and involvement in the learning process are strengthened
  3.5 Direct learners to the literature and other resources when they lack prerequisite knowledge or have special interests
  3.6 Assign outside reading or tasks to reinforce learning
  3.7 Describe differences between inpatient and outpatient teaching
  3.8 Orient learners to each particular patient care setting
  3.9 Help learners set realistic learning expectations by assigning responsibilities appropriate to the developmental stage of each learner
  3.10 Insert oneself into the clinical situation to model appropriate practices, attitudes, and interpersonal skills

GOAL 5.0: Assess student performance

  5.1 Identify different purposes for evaluating performance such as diagnosing learning, assigning grades, and certifying learners
  5.2 Use checklists and rating scales when observing live or recorded learner performance
  5.3 Keep anecdotal records to evaluate learner progress
  5.4 Give learner positive and negative feedback on progress toward achieving course/program objectives
  5.5 Counsel learners to help them develop self-evaluation skills
  5.6 Understand various mechanisms for evaluating learner progress and choose a method appropriate for a given purpose
  5.7 Use simulations including print, computer, patients, and videotape
  5.8 Design and conduct oral examinations
  5.9 Conduct and interpret simple checks on reliability and validity of evaluation methods
  5.10 Design written tests that include objective short answer and essay type questions

Research

GOAL 11.0: Access and critically read the research literature in medicine, education, and other domains

  11.1 Use appropriate resources (libraries, computers) to complete literature searches
  11.2 Evaluate a research article critically

References

Bergquist, W. H., & Phillips, S. R. (1975). Components of an effective faculty development program. *Journal of Higher Education, 46*, 177–209.

Blackburn, R. T. (1979). Academic careers: Patterns and possibilities. *Current Issues in Higher Education, 2*, 25–27.

Bland, C. J., Hitchcock, M., Anderson, W., & Stritter, F. T. (1986, March 4). *Study of graduates of family medicine faculty development fellowship programs. Final report from the Society for Teachers for Family Medicine (STFM) Task Force on Faculty Development* (HRSA Contract #84 592(p), Final Report). Rockville, MD: Health and Human Services Administration, Division of Medicine.

Bland, C. J., Hitchcock, M. A., Anderson, W. A., & Stritter, F. T. (1987, August). Faculty development fellowship programs in family medicine. *Journal of Medical Education, 62*(8), 632–641.

Bland, C. J., & Schmitz, C. C., (1986). Characteristics of the successful researcher and implications for faculty development. Journal of Medical Education, 61, 22–31.

Bland, C. J., & Schmitz, C. C., (1988). Faculty vitality on review: Retrospect and prospect. *Journal of Higher Education, 59*, 191–224.

Corcoran, M., & Clark, S. M., (1984). Professional socialization and contemporary career attitudes of three faculty generations. *Research in Higher Education, 20*(2), 131–153.

Gaff, J. G. (1976). *Toward faculty renewal.* San Francisco: Jossey-Bass.

Houle, C. O. (1980). *Continuing learning in the professions.* San Francisco: Jossey-Bass.

Katz, R. L. (1978). Job longevity as a situational factor in job satisfaction. *Administrative Science Quarterly, 23*, 204–223.

McGaghie, W. C., & Frey, J. J. (Eds.). (1986). *Handbook for the academic physician.* New York: Springer-Verlag.

Perkoff, G. T. (1985, November). The research environment in family practice. *Journal of Family Practice, 21*(5), 389–393.

Schuster, J. H., & Wheeler, D. W. (in press). *Enhancing faculty careers: Strategies for renewal.* San Francisco: Jossey-Bass.

Sherman, C. (1983, December 14). *Percentage of MD postdoctoral trainees who applied for and received a grant, by length of supported training* (table). Presentation at the 48th meeting of the Advisory Committee to the Director of National Institutes of Health, Bethesda, Maryland.

Tyler, R. W. (1950). *Basic principles of curriculum and instruction.* Chicago: University of Chicago.

CHAPTER 3

Education Domain

Introduction to the Domain

For many medical faculty members, clinical teaching represents the most important aspect of their jobs. Most primary care faculty spend as much as 30% of their time in teaching—it is the heart of what a faculty career means. Whether faculty members chose that career before, after, or in addition to a medical practice, they probably did so because they aspired to teach. Interestingly, the Latin verb "docere," meaning to teach, is also the root for the noun "doctor." It seems that the doctor who teaches, then, comes by that function quite appropriately.

Once in academic medicine, the physician faculty member learns that teaching is only one task within the broader domain of education, but it usually remains the central one. The faculty member also learns that teaching is challenging. Medical students and residents provide medical care for their patients while they learn from them. Somehow, clinical teachers must integrate their responsibilities for those patients and their right to competent care with the demands of instruction and the learner's need to learn. Fortunately, a body of knowledge does exist to help faculty balance these responsibilities.

Definition of the Domain

Education in the health professions has its roots in the academic disciplines of education and psychology. Although the practice of medical teaching is as old as Hippocrates, modern medical education is closely tied to the academic foundations of teaching, learning, and adult education. Medical teaching is facilitated by a systematic

approach to instruction and by emerging research on medical education and on clinical teaching. Like its cousins, elementary, secondary,
and college education, medical education includes the broad range
of tasks associated with curriculum design and development, teaching, student assessment, and program evaluation. Medical faculty
spend much of their teaching time engaged directly with learners,
delivering instruction. Much less time, proportionally speaking, is
spent planning or evaluating curricula. Thus, this component draws
more deeply from the research on teaching in general, and on clinical teaching specifically.

The literature has been helpful in developing this component.
For example, Rosenshine and Stevens (1986) summarized the more
important research on teaching by reviewing effective classroom
instructors at a variety of educational levels. They concluded that effective teachers generally accomplish certain events of instruction. Those
events are to: (1) begin a session with a short review of previous,
prerequisite learning, (2) follow with a short statement of goals for
the session, (3) present new material in relatively short steps with
learner practice after each step, (4) give clear and detailed explana-
tions, (5) ask many questions and obtain responses from all learners,
(6) guide learners during initial practice, (7) provide a high level of
successful practice, and (8) provide systematic feedback and constructive criticism to each learner.

It is difficult to apply these steps to an apprenticeship (a major
teaching strategy to medical education) as strictly as one can in classroom teaching, simply because the stimulus for teaching and learning in clinical encounters is more spontaneous. Often the stimulus
is an unpredictable encounter with a patient, the nature and content
of which cannot be planned. Still, a recent review of studies on clinical instruction (Dinham & Stritter, 1986) found that effective clinical instructors perform tasks similar to those listed above. Effective
clinical teachers (1) organize learning by providing clear direction,
goals, expectations, and criteria for completion, (2) provide guided practice and evaluation of performance, (3) display interest in the learner
and enthusiasm for teaching, and (4) provide competent role models
of the profession to which the students aspire.

Support for competencies in this domain comes from researchers
in nonmedical education, such as Rosenshine and Stevens (1986), and
medical education, such as Dinham and Stritter (1986). Additional
research supporting the clinical instruction competencies has been
done by Gil, Heins, and Jones (1984), Irby (1978), Mattern, Weinholtz,
and Friedman (1983), and Stritter and Baker (1982). Curricular content and development in medical education has been addressed by

Eichna (1983), Friedman, Slatt, Baker, and Cummings (1983), Guilbert (1984), and Harden (1984). Learner and program evaluation in medical education have been well delineated by Bland, Ullian, and Froberg (1984), Irby (1983), McGuire (1983), Petrusa (1984), and Skeff, Campbell, and Stratos (1984).

Recurring throughout this literature and the related competencies is the view that education seeks to change learners' attitudes and behaviors in some constructive and largely predetermined manner. To accomplish this, the events of instruction should be structured and approached as systematically as possible, for program planning, teaching, and evaluation are essentially interactive in nature.

The effective clinical instructor, then, applies systematic principles of teaching found effective in general education settings, while functioning as a professional role model at the same time. Accordingly, the competencies in Education stress the systematic steps of instruction as they apply to curriculum development and teaching in clinical settings.

Rationale for Including Education in the Curriculum

Although teaching has long been recognized as a critical (perhaps the initial and most basic) domain in faculty development, new faculty often tend to underestimate the skill and time it takes to plan courses, prepare lectures, advise students, lead seminars, and evaluate programs. On a daily basis, faculty members will find that the skills of curriculum planning, teaching, and evaluation will enable them to carry out their teaching responsibilities more effectively.

How the Domain Has Been Structured

The domain has been structured according to the major subareas of knowledge undergirding effective instruction (see Figure 3.1 below). These areas imply a sequence to the process of planning educational programs, designing instruction, teaching, and evaluating learners and educational programs.

Five premises characterize this structure. First, the goal of any instructional program is to change learner attitudes and/or behaviors in a predetermined direction. To do this the instructor must focus on what the learner does during instruction; this differs from traditional views of instruction, which tend to focus on what the instructor does and the content that the instructor covers in an encounter. Second, these subareas represent interdependent components. Each component (i.e., program planning, teaching, and evaluation) has a specific

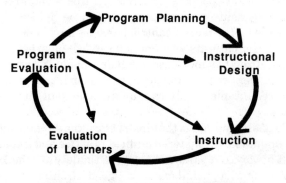

FIGURE 3.1 The education domain.

function, but they interact with one another so that change in one is likely to affect the entire plan. Third, accomplishing the components provides a basis for sequential decisions. They do not always have to be addressed in the sequence shown above, but none is adequate if addressed alone. Fourth, programs and teaching can be improved over time through successive waves of implementation, evaluation, and revision. A systematic approach does not guarantee an optimal program the first time it is taught, although its use does increase chances of a successful initial effort. The approach does, however, virtually guarantee improvement over time. Since many programs are taught over and over again, often by the same instructor, gradual improvement becomes possible. Fifth, as mentioned, medical faculty spend most of their teaching time engaged directly with learners. For this reason, the domain is weighted heavily in the teaching area. Competencies, courses, and teaching strategies are greater in number and detail in teaching than they are in other areas (e.g., program planning, evaluation).

Assumptions Made in Constructing the Domain

There are three assumptions upon which this domain is based. The first and most important is that learning must be planned. It will not happen spontaneously; it cannot be left to chance. Even though each student's or resident's clinical experience will be different and the learning encounters somewhat unpredictable, teachers still need to provide structure. They need to clearly understand the goals of instruction and the competencies they wish to impart. They need to have an arsenal of teaching strategies to draw from in order to capitalize on a teachable event.

A second assumption is that within this structured learning environment students and residents should be helped to learn for themselves. Given the lack of control teachers have over the learning environment, the patients who enter it, and the learners when they are not being directly supervised, such autonomy is critical. Only by increasing learners' responsibility for their own learning and by holding them accountable for it can an independent professional be educated.

The final assumption is that instructors know their content areas well. They should have mastered clinical practice and have conceptualized it in a way that allows them to articulate it when teaching. Without this knowledge and expertise, good teaching is not possible.

The old adage, "teachers are born, not made," is a misconception that hinders both the faculty members who try to teach without adequate preparation and those who devote many hours to planning and developing their teaching. This domain has been designed with the belief that teaching skills, as well as the skills of planning and practice, can be learned. Becoming familiar with the approach described here should give faculty the knowledge, skills, and confidence to develop their individual teaching abilities and styles.

Goals and Competencies

Listed below are the goals and competencies for the Education domain. This list represents the full spectrum of knowledge and skills required of medical faculty in Education. It is not broken down by institution or faculty type. For suggestions on how to identify relevant competencies for preceptors, non-tenure-track, and tenure-track faculty, see Chapter 2.

Program Planning

GOAL 1.0: To design educational programs (curricula) with appropriate scope, sequence, and focus for intended learners.

Program planning involves all the planning that is done in order to set up an educational program or curriculum. Typically, planning decisions involve the assessment of a given educational setting (e.g., the institutional mission, the department's goals, the resources and facilities available for teaching) and an identified group of learners (e.g., characteristics and needs of students, residents, fellows, or faculty). Once these factors have been analyzed, instructors can map out the curriculum to be covered and subdivide the content into appropriate units, rotations, or courses.

Faculty should be able to:

1.1. Articulate a program purpose
1.2. Identify salient characteristics of potential participants (e.g., amount of previous learning)
1.3. Research and synthesize literature relevant to program topics
1.4. Evaluate instructional resources and constraints by analyzing the environment
1.5. Select and sequence curricular content
1.6. Write program goals

Instructional Design

GOAL 2.0: To develop courses, presentations, and course materials using a systematic approach.

Instructional design includes those tasks associated with planning a rotation, course, or seminar. To begin this process, faculty members write objectives that explain what learners should be able to know, do, or feel as a result of instruction. Objectives can vary in specificity, but they serve as a planning tool, a guide for learners, a form of communication between teachers, and a basis for evaluation. After preparing objectives, faculty members select teaching strategies that are appropriate. To prepare these strategies, faculty research and screen existing instructional materials or prepare their own.

Faculty should be able to:

2.1. Translate broad educational goals into specific instructional objectives
2.2. Classify objectives according to types of learning required (i.e., verbal skills, intellectual skills, problem-solving skills, motor skills, and attitudes)
2.3. Develop instructional units (i.e., segments that can be undertaken by learners at one time) from objectives
2.4. Choose a teaching format (e.g., course readings, preceptorship) appropriate for the instructional purpose

2.5. Apply general principles of adult learning (e.g., set expectations, practice opportunities, evaluate performance, provide feedback)

2.6. Plan individual sessions, including teaching strategies to be used (e.g., lecture, small group)

2.7. Select or prepare instructional resources and materials syllabi, visuals

Teaching

GOAL 3.0: To teach individuals and small groups in clinic and at bedside.

GOAL 4.0: To deliver instruction to small and large groups in classroom settings, using a variety of strategies.

Instructional strategies encompass the actual skills of teaching. They include techniques that instructors use to present and reinforce information, stimulate thinking, and trigger discussion and synthesis. These techniques vary somewhat, depending on the format (e.g., lecture, small group, seminar) being used. One additional technique that instructors should develop is the ability to improvise—to respond rapidly to a variety of events, unforeseen opportunities, questions raised by learners, and other occurrences (e.g., "teachable moments") that are totally unplanned—particularly as they relate to situations provided by patients.

Faculty should be able to:

General

3.1. Clearly explain course objectives and directions to learners

3.2. Help learners organize their learning activities

3.3. Ask questions at various taxonomic levels to stimulate thinking

3.4. Respond to learners so that their interest and involvement in the learning process are strengthened

3.5. Direct learners to the literature and other resources when they lack prerequisite knowledge or have special interests

3.6. Assign outside readings or tasks to reinforce learning

Clinical Instruction

3.7. Describe differences between inpatient and outpatient teaching

3.8. Orient learners to each particular patient care setting

3.9. Help learners set realistic learning expectations by assigning responsibilities appropriate to the developmental stage of each learner

3.10. Insert oneself into the clinical situation to model appropriate practices, attitudes, and interpersonal skills

Large Group Instruction

4.1. Research a topic and gather materials for a lecture

4.2. Prepare a written outline for a lecture

4.3. Deliver a lecture that includes the use of audiovisuals, follow-up questions, and discussion

Small Group Instruction

4.4. Coordinate various types of small group instruction (e.g., seminars, simulations, discussions)

4.5. Develop tasks and/or problems to be addressed by a group

4.6. Lead a discussion and delegate tasks to group members

4.7. Develop simulations to be used by a group

Evaluation of the Learner

GOAL 5.0: To assess student performance.

To assess how much students or residents have learned, faculty need to understand the overall purpose(s) of evaluation. They should be familiar with a range of assessment methods and be able to choose an appropriate method given the purpose at hand. Evaluation should be based directly on the objectives and help both the instructor and the learner to determine if objectives have been met. Selecting or developing an approach to evaluation should be accomplished soon after the objectives have been determined, and occasionally even prior to writing objectives. In addition, the instructor must be able to implement each method and communicate the results to learners in the form of feedback.

Faculty should be able to:

5.1. Identify different purposes for evaluating performance such as diagnosing learning, assigning grades, and certifying learners

5.2. Use checklists and rating scales when observing live or recorded learner performance

5.3. Keep anecdotal records to evaluate learner progress

5.4. Give learner positive and negative feedback on progress toward achieving course/program objectives

5.5. Counsel learners to help them develop self-evaluation skills

5.6. Understand various mechanisms for evaluating learner progress and choose a method appropriate for a given purpose

5.7. Use simulations including print, computer, patients, and videotape

5.8. Design and conduct oral examinations

5.9. Conduct and interpret simple checks on reliability and validity of evaluation methods

5.10. Design written tests that include objective, short answer and essay-type questions

Evaluation of Education Programs

GOAL 6.0: To evaluate program effectiveness both formatively and summatively.

To evaluate the effectiveness of programs and instruction, faculty need to make empirical judgments concerning their quality. Judgment is based on evaluation. Evaluation involves identifying program purposes, collecting and interpreting data, and reporting judgments based on the conclusions. After making judgments, instruction should be revised to incorporate the indicated changes.

Faculty should be able to:

6.1. Identify questions, the answers to which will inform specific decisions about the instructional program

6.2. Develop an evaluation plan to include a data collection instrument(s) (e.g., questionnaire, interview, test)

6.3. Determine the most appropriate data source(s) (e.g., self, learners, peers, administrators, and/or experts) and collect the data

6.4. Analyze the data and interpret the results

6.5. Report results to concerned individuals

6.6. Revise instruction as appropriate

Courses, Strategies, and Resources

Described below are the suggested courses, strategies, and resources for teaching the competencies and achieving the goals of the Education domain. (Competencies to be achieved by each course or activity are listed by number after each description.) These activities and sources cover the full range of skills identified for Education; they are not keyed to specific faculty types at particular institutions. For guidelines on how to select and combine courses in this and other domains for preceptors, non-tenure-track, and tenure-track faculty, see Chapter 8.

101. CLINICAL INSTRUCTION (Six 4-hour sessions)

This series of workshops is designed to help clinical instructors become sensitive to the considerations involved in one-on-one clinic or bedside teaching. The significant events of clinical instruction include setting expectations for learners, arranging clinical experiences and presentations, asking questions that stimulate clinical reasoning skills, evaluating performance, and providing feedback to learners. All of these events are implemented differently depending on the stage of development reached by the learner at the time of the instruction.

Strategies

1. Participants identify perceived strengths and weaknesses of their own clinical teaching or of teaching they have experienced. The discussion leader lists those identified on a blackboard and comments briefly on them. This is a good discussion starter.
2. Participants take and score Attitudes Toward Increasing Learner Responsibility Inventory (ATILR) [available in Stritter, Baker, & Shahady (1986)]. The leader discusses variance in scores by relating them to variance in learners' stages of development.
3. In a small group discussion format, present and discuss the "Learning Vector" model for clinical instruction (Stritter et al., 1986).
4. Participants take and score "The clinical learner: A consensus exercise on resident preferences for clinical teaching" (Stritter et al., 1986), then discuss it in small groups to arrive at agreement. The leader discusses differences between groups and residents' actual view of teaching.

5. Participants view an 8- to 10-minute videotape or simulation of a one-on-one precipitating encounter or chart
   review. Participants discuss, "What did you see happen-
   ing or not that should have?" The leader lists principles
   of clinical teaching that emerge. This list is refined until
   the group is satisfied that the list of 8 to 10 principles
   can be used to guide and evaluate clinical teaching.
   Leaders can indicate how the self-generated list correlates with research on the topic, but items should come
   from participants.
6. The criteria for evaluating clinical teaching (agreed
   upon in above) are used to analyze and evaluate three
   additional 4- to 5-minute videotapes, each depicting
   another aspect of encounters with learners. Examples
   of aspects to evaluate could include the setting of expectations with the learner, questioning, or providing feedback. At the end of the discussion, criteria are again
   reviewed to determine if they are appropriate.
7. Participants divide into groups of three to practice
   aspects of clinical teaching based on criteria. Participants practice, observe, critique, and discuss case
   studies while the leader facilitates the process. Sample
   case studies and processes are described in Stritter et
   al., (1986).
8. Participants are assigned the task of completing one live
   videotape of a teaching incident with a medical student
   or resident. The tape should be no more than 10 minutes
   long and focus on one or two criteria of clinical teaching specified by each participant in advance. In reviewing tapes, participants are asked to indicate: (1) stage
   of learner's development, (2) self-perception of teaching
   effectiveness based on aspect(s) specified, and (3) other
   aspects that now require further work. Tapes are reviewed in groups of four, with discussion facilitated by
   a leader. Additional tapes can be reviewed in subsequent
   sessions, with each participant focusing on a different
   criterion during each review.

Suggested Topics

• Staged development of a learner
• Diagnosis of learner's needs
• Characteristics of effective clinical teaching

- Setting expectations and performance criteria with learners
- Roles and responsibilities of learners (e.g., case presentations)
- Questioning skills
- Evaluation and feedback
- Arriving at closure

Competencies: 3.1 through 3.10; 5.1, 5.3, 5.4, and 5.5.

Suggested Resource Material

Edwards, J. C., & Marier, R. L. (1988). *Clinical teaching for medical residents: Roles, techniques, and programs.* Focuses on teaching residents how to teach, but discusses several generic approaches to teaching that are worthwhile.

Ende, J. (1983). Feedback in clinical medical education. A good discussion of feedback techniques.

Irby, D. M. (1986). Clinical teaching and the clinical teacher.

Pratt, D., & McGill, M. (1983). Educational contracts: A basis for effective clinical teaching. A nice rationale for and approach to setting expectations with learners.

Schwenk, T. L., & Whitman, N. (1987). *The physician as teacher.* An excellent review of the many aspects of clinical teaching, including a chapter on ambulatory teaching.

Stritter, F., Baker, R., & Shahady, E. (1986). Clinical instruction. In W. C. McGaghie & J. J. Frey (Eds.), *Handbook for the academic physician.* Several useful exercises and discussions.

Stritter, F., & Flair, M. (1980). *Effective clinical teaching.* Provides an overview of the entire process of clinical teaching.

Weinholz, D. (1983). Directing medical student client case presentations. Discusses the utility of different question types in clinical teaching.

102. A CURRICULUM PLANNING MODEL (Four 4-hour sessions)

These sessions are designed to assist instructors in planning courses and other educational programs. A flexible model is suggested that offers instructors an approach to making important decisions about courses. The model suggests a modified role for the instructor, that of manager of an instructional program rather than a conveyor of information.

Strategies

1. Participants begin by identifying what they believe to be the main organizational characteristics of the most and

least effective educational programs they have known. The leader lists characteristics on the blackboard and uses the list as a basis for discussion.

2. Leaders present and facilitate discussion on the "systematic approach" model for program design. A short 35mm slide program can be used to highlight and illustrate decision making in such a model (Stritter & Howell, 1983). It is often helpful to present an example of a program that has been designed using the systems model.

3. Participants can analyze a brief case study describing the development of an instructional program. A residency program can provide appropriate material for such a case study. Participants review the case, then indicate what was done to address each of the steps in the planning model, and finally indicate what the participants would have advised the planning committee to do. Individual participants or small groups can analyze the case.

4. Participants can be divided into groups of four to develop the curriculum for a residency program based on a "Mother Nature" strategy (Friedman & Baker, 1986). This provides participants with practical experience in collecting information on which to base their planning decisions.

5. Each participant is asked to develop the outline of an educational program for which he is responsible. A workbook can be used to walk participants through a planning process. Feedback can come either from the leader or from fellow participants after a presentation and review of the program outline are developed. Participants can often work effectively in pairs to accomplish the review and feedback process.

Suggested Topics

• Defining educationally relevant topics to address (e.g., a community health problem)
• Developing broad goals
• Ascertaining program context
• Selecting and sequencing concepts to be taught
• Writing instructional objectives
• Preparing approaches for assessment

- Outlining each concept
- Implementing a program
- Evaluating a program
- Revising a program

Competencies: 1.1 through 1.6, and 2.1 through 2.7.

Suggested Resource Material

Bandaranayake, R. C. (1986). *How to plan a medical curriculum.* Helpful approach to educational planning.
Foley, R. P. & Smilansky, J. (1980). Instructional design. In *Teaching techniques: A handbook for health professionals.* Presents a good analytic plan from which an individualized exercise could be developed.
Friedman, C. P., & Baker, R. M. (1986). An experience in curriculum development. In W. C. McGaghie & J. J. Frey (Eds.), *Handbook for the academic physician.* Contains a good group exercise in planning a curriculum.
Stritter, F. T., & Bowles, L. T. (1972). *The teacher as manager: A strategy for medical education.* Outlines an efficient and effective systematic approach to instruction.
Stritter, F. T., & Howell, B. (1983). *A systematic approach to instruction* (a 35mm slide program). Illustrates a sound instructional planning model.

103. LEARNING PRINCIPLES AND INSTRUCTIONAL OBJECTIVES (One or two 4-hour sessions)

Learning theory and research on learning can be helpful in indicating how people learn best and in creating conditions that maximize the achievement of instructional objectives by learners. Medical students and residents are adults; therefore, guidelines from the literature on adult learning theory are appropriate. When applying general learning principles, instructors should realize that each learner has different educational experiences and personality characteristics that influence learning. They should also know what those principles are and how they can be used in planning instruction.

Based on learning theory and the information, concepts, or skills to be learned, instructional objectives can be developed for each unit of instruction. Those objectives assist the instructor in planning, guide the learner in approaching a complex learning task, and communicate intentions to fellow instructors. Objectives can be developed in different ways as no single approach has been uniformly effective. A simple approach is best—one that states what learners should be able to know, do, or feel as a result of instruction.

Strategies

1. Participants can assess their own learning style with various instruments, such as the Rezler Learning Preference Inventory (Foley & Smilansky, 1980) or the Kolb Learning Style Inventory (Kolb, 1984). Results can be used as a basis of discussion.

2. Use a presentation and discussion format to present the principles of learning and the types of objectives. A 35mm slide program or overhead transparencies emphasizing key points can illustrate a presentation.

3. Participants can be given a checklist of learning principles and asked to individually analyze a course, program, or workshop in which they have recently been a participant, either as a learner or an instructor. This can be revised as a group exercise by using a written case study to analyze and discuss.

4. Participants can develop a list of the learning principles for their own course/program indicating how they will attend to each principle. This can be reviewed by the leader or by other members of the group organized in pairs.

5. Readings about instructional objectives (e.g., Kibler, Cegala, Watson, Barker, & Miles, 1981) should be assigned as preparation for a lecture/discussion. A presentation using audiovisual materials can emphasize the taxonomies, levels, and uses of objectives. An excessive amount of detail about the complexities of objectives can, however, hinder a discussion.

6. Exercises in which objectives are classified and revised either individually or in groups are a useful strategy. The exercises should be prepared in advance and used as a self-assessment or as the basis for group discussion.

7. Participants can also develop goals and/or objectives for their own teaching, then review and critique each other's list.

Suggested Topics

• Meaningfulness of objectives and content
• Prerequisites to be met by learners

- Modeling of skills and concepts to be learned
- Open communication between learners and instructors
- Practice of concepts/skills to be learned
- Reinforcement/feedback as a principle of learning
- The taxonomies of cognitive and affective objectives
- Use of objectives

Competencies: 1.2, 1.6, 2.3, 2.4, 2.5, 3.2, and 3.3.

Suggested Resource Material

Bonner, J. (1982). Systematic lesson design for adult learners. Covers adult learning principles as they are applied to course design.

Davis, R. H., Alexander, F. T., & Yelon, S. L. (1975). General principles of learning and motivation. In *Learning system design: An approach to the improvement of instruction.* Presents a simple but effective explanation of learning principles.

Kibler, R. L., Cegala, D. J., Watson, K. W. Barker, L. L., & Miles, D. T. (1981). *Objectives for instruction and evaluation.* Currently out of print, but an excellent resource for learning about objectives.

Knowles, M. S. (1978). *The adult learner: A neglected species.* A classic, but still useful.

104. LARGE GROUP PRESENTATIONS (Two or three 4-hour sessions)

The effective lecture is the sine qua non of higher education, but its purpose is limited in the clinical component of medical education. A large group presentation is one in which an instructor addresses 15 learners or more, and in which interaction with participants is minimal. A lecture is effective for efficiently presenting information to learners. It can provide up-to-date information, synthesize large bodies of information from multiple sources, help learners build a framework for further study, and communicate an instructor's enthusiasm for and expertise in a topic.

Strategies

1. Use a lecture and discussion format to present the principles and components of oral presentations. This should be brief, well-planned, and rehearsed to serve as a model for the participants. The leader should convey that a good lecture is well-organized and includes a rousing introduction and an outline of key points to be covered.

A good lecture has a cogent, well-paced body of information supported by visual illustrations where appropriate. It should not require learners to be attentive for long periods (i.e., more than an hour). It includes various concrete examples, active learner participation when possible, thought-provoking questions, and a concise explanation of key concepts. Finally, it includes specific conclusions that summarize principal points, reiterate the framework, and encourage questions from learners.

2. Participants should prepare and present short (3- to 5-minute) introductions to lectures to the group. The introduction can be constructively critiqued by the group as a starting point for discussion.
3. Participants should then list criteria by which they will develop and evaluate presentations. This is accomplished after the first set of mini-presentations has been completed.
4. A series of videotapes can be developed, each depicting a different aspect of a lecture. The tapes can then be used for analysis with participants critiquing each of the various aspects. The tapes can be real or simulated; they can be ideal or problem situations. Problem situations often lead to creative problem-solving by participants.
5. Microteaching is an invaluable method for improving lecture skills. Participants present portions of their lectures (e.g., introductions or conclusions), have them videotaped, and then review them using the list of criteria developed above. Fellow participants can provide constructive criticism. This procedure can be followed several times, focusing on a different aspect for the presentation each time.

Suggested Tasks

• Organizing lecture material, principal themes, and concepts
• The introduction
• Learners' retention strategies
• Learner participation
• Audiovisual support
• Summary and conclusion

Competencies: 3.1 through 3.6, and 4.1 through 4.3.

Suggested Resource Material

Abrahamson, S., & Wilkow, M. (1984). *The lecture: A problem solving unit.* A 35mm slide-illustrated instructional program.

Cashin, W., & McKnight, P. C. (1985). *Improving lectures.* Provides best brief guide to presenting better large group presentations.

Cox, K. R., & Ewan, C. E. (1988). *The medical teacher.* Contains excellent suggestions in a brief overview.

Foley, R. P., & Smilansky, J. (1980). The lecture. In *Teaching techniques: A handbook for health professionals.* An excellent discussion of a lecture's characteristics.

105. SMALL GROUP TEACHING (Two to three 4-hour sessions)

Medical teachers have many opportunities to teach in small groups. A small group includes 3 to 13 learners and can be convened either with or without an instructor. In seminars, faculty typically give brief lecturettes and then interact with learners in a question-and-answer format. A teacher also organizes attending rounds, in which 3 to 6 learners at different stages of their development participate, each having a different responsibility for the patient being discussed. A teacher can also structure small learner-centered groups and act as a consultant rather than participate actively in the group. Groups can be assigned the task of analyzing some entity, solving a problem or participating in a role play. In this case, the teacher develops the task, encourages the group to respond to the task on its own, and then helps the group to process and understand its response.

Strategies

1. Ask learners to read selected references from the resource section prior to attending the session. First spend a little time discussing the concepts of small group learning, then proceed directly into experiential learning by asking participants to be involved in group exercises of the type being taught. A videotape of a group interaction can also provide the stimulus for discussion, but there are advantages to having participants create and use their own group. Leaders should emphasize the multiple functions that groups can serve, such as providing the instructor with feedback on what and how learners understand; assisting in accomplishing higher-level cognitive goals; helping learners develop interests,

values, and attitudes; and allowing learners to become active participants in their own learning.

2. Develop two to three exercises in which the group can participate immediately. One could be a 20-minute seminar led by the instructor and based on the reading, another a 20-minute clinical problem to analyze or solve and/or a 20-minute role play on a health policy issue. The leader would lead the first, observe only in the second, and participate as a group member in the third. At the end of the hour, participants would construct a list of 10 criteria by which they could analyze learning groups.

3. Participants would observe three different 10-minute videotapes of actual learning groups to determine the degree to which the criteria had been met. The leader would lead a discussion modeling the criteria.

4. Each participant would be asked to design a seminar or group exercise of his own and then to conduct it in simulated fashion using other members of the group as his learners. The interactions should be approximately 15 minutes each.

5. Each participant could videotape his own seminar or attending round and bring it back to the group for analysis. This can be done more than once.

Suggested Topics

- Objectives that can be accomplished in a group
- Behaviors of group members
- Structuring a group but feeling comfortable with less control
- Setting the environment for learning
- Integrating content into discussion

Competencies: 3.1 through 3.6, and 4.4 through 4.7.

Suggested Resource Material

Cashin, W. E., & McKnight, P. C. (1986). *Improving discussions.* Provides excellent guidance for leading seminars.

Cox, K. R., & Ewan, C. E. (1988). *The medical teacher.* A brief but useful guide written especially for the physician.

Mattern, W., Weinholtz, D., & Friedman, C. (1983). The attending physician as teacher. Contains a particularly good perspective for the attending physician who conducts teaching rounds with medical students and residents.

Olmstead, J. A. (1979). *Small group instruction: Theory and practice.* Good information on several types of small group exercises.

Whitman, N. A., Swhwenk, T. L. (1983). *A handbook for group discussion leaders: Alternatives to lecturing students to death.* A very practical and simple guidebook.

106. SELECTION AND USE OF INSTRUCTIONAL MEDIA
(One to two 4-hour sessions)

The term *media* incorporates all methods that an instructor uses to communicate an instructional message to learners. Media can be as simple as an overhead projector or as complex as a videodisc. Media can be used to present a stimulus, illustrate a point, elicit a response from learners, or provide feedback to learners.

Participants should be taught that a few simple rules can guide choices about which media to use: (1) base the selection on course objectives, (2) select the simplest possible medium, and (3) use more than one medium whenever possible to reinforce important points.

Strategies

1. Use lecture, demonstration, and discussion to illustrate a selected number of media types and uses.
2. Using an evaluation form that includes specific criteria, evaluate one or two media for validity, utility, and feasibility, and follow up with a discussion of the process.
3. A media fair can be useful in which participants receive hands-on experience with a small number of media. Participants could preview model slide programs, videotapes, and computer software.
4. Have participants take a series of slides for use in a presentation. Have them describe their objectives, intended audience, and purpose of the slides. They might also prepare a set of transparencies or a videotape and then give a short presentation.
5. Ask participants to discuss how the computer might be used as an instructional tool. Develop a situation in which participants would use computer-based materials. Include a description of learners, the objectives, the role of the computer, and anticipated learner outcomes using the computer.

6. Ask participants to develop or choose one media presentation, use it in their actual instruction, and report results to the group.

Suggested Topics

- Types of media
- Advantages and disadvantages of various types of media
- Selecting media
- Designing simple media
- Evaluating available media
- Using media

Competencies: 2.4 and 4.3.

Suggested Resource Material

Abrahamson, S., Wilkow, M., & Bartenstein, S. (1984). *The use of media.* A 35mm slide-illustrated instructional program.
Beery, M. P. (1986). Visuals for oral and written presentations. In W. C. McGaghie & J. J. Frey (Eds.), *Handbook for the academic physician.* Contains brief but helpful description of using media.
Cox, K. R., & Ewan, C. E. (1988). *The medical teacher.* This is a practical guide for any clinical teacher.
Heinrich, R., Molenda, M., & Russell, J. D. (1985). *Instructional media and the new technologies of instruction.* This book is written with much detail and must be used selectively, but it covers the complete range of possibilities available to the instructor.

107. ASSESSMENT OF LEARNERS (Two or three 4-hour sessions)

Leaders should emphasize that learners in any educational program are evaluated for several purposes. First, assessment exercises can give the learner practice in using the content taught in a program followed by feedback about the adequacy of performance. Second, assessment can assist in making decisions about learner competencies. Learners studying medical topics and skills must be certified as to their competence before moving to a subsequent level or being allowed to practice. Third, assessment can help in selecting participants for the next level of study. Finally, assessment of learners can provide an index of whether or not an educational program is accomplishing its purpose. If several learners are not able to demonstrate the knowledge or skill taught in the program, then the program has problems that must be remedied. Participants should understand that assessment is critical, as it communicates subtle messages concerning what is important for learners to derive from the educational program. The most elegantly designed and delivered presentation will not likely be well-remembered unless it is also tested in some way. The assessment of learners in a curriculum, is, in essence, the "hidden" curriculum.

Participants should also be taught how the science of measurement facilitates assessment. This science helps instructors decide what to assess (e.g., knowledge, skills, attitudes), how to assess (e.g., objective written lists, oral examinations, observations of performance in simulated or actual patient encounters, review of records), what the criteria are, how to set standards, how to ensure that the data obtained have quality, and how to compare performance to a norm, a standard, or some combination of the two.

Strategies

1. Participants read basic readings selected from resources and then participate in a lecture/discussion based on the principal issues of measurement and evaluation. Included in the presentation should be contemporary types of assessment, such as standardized or simulated patients, role playing, oral examination, patient management problems, and modified essay questions.
2. Participants develop a test plan for the educational program they are evaluating (e.g., a clerkship, a rotation, a course, or a year-long program). The test plan should include objectives to be evaluated, methods for evaluating each objective, and samples of specific items.
3. Participants develop all or part of selected instruments (e.g., a written test, a clinical problem, a rating scale, or a checklist) that they are using as part of their test plan. The instruments should be reviewed and critiqued by fellow participants for technique and validity.
4. A videotape of clinical performance can be reviewed using a rating scale developed either by the group or by the leader. This can help establish interrater reliability and sensitize participants to the need for rater training in evaluation.
5. Participants review either simulated item analysis data, developed by the leader, or actual data gathered by their

own instrument, to understand the purpose of reviewing exam statistics.

6. Participants can construct components of an Objective Structured Clinical Exam (OSCE), a multi-station differentiated evaluation, for medical students or residents (Harden, Stevenson, Downle, & Wilson, 1975). This can be undertaken in groups and results can then be pooled.

Suggested Topics

• Criterion versus norm-referenced measurement
• Item analysis (e.g., discrimination index, difficulty index)
• Reliability
• Validity
• Standard error of measurement
• Variety of techniques available, such as simulated patients, role plays, oral exams, and patient management problems
• Objective Structure Clinical Exam (OSCE)

Competencies: 5.1–5.3 and 5.6–5.10.

Suggested Resource Material

Harden, M., Stevenson, M., Downle, W. V. & Wilson, G. M. (1975). Assessment of clinical competence using the objective structured clinical examination. An initial discussion of a comprehensive approach to reviewing clinical performance.

McGaghie, W. (1986). Evaluation of learners. In W. C. McGaghie & J. J. Frey (Eds.), *Handbook for the academic physician*. A brief but effective review of major measurement considerations.

Morgan, M. K., & Irby, D. M. (Eds.). (1978). *Evaluating clinical competencies in the health professions.* A systematic review of all approaches useful in evaluating clinical competence.

Nuefeld, V. R., & Norman, G. R. (1985). *Assessing clinical competence.* A description of all the approaches used at McMaster University. Includes a good review of the literature.

Popham, W. J. (1981). *Modern educational measurement.* An introductory text on educational testing that simply and briefly discusses important measurement concepts such as validity and reliability.

108. EVALUATION OF PROGRAMS (Two 4-hour sessions)

In this course the leader should define program evaluation as the process of systematically collecting information about one or more educational program issues and reporting it in a form that allows those responsible to make decisions about the program. Such information can be provided to faculty to enable them to change the way instruction is organized and delivered; it can also be provided to administrators to justify or eliminate current programs or practices.

Participants should understand that evaluation is a process that should occur throughout an educational program, either formally with an instrument of some type, or informally by merely observing or talking with participants. Faculty should emphasize that (1) a grade or similar symbol is not useful evaluation data unless a learner can employ it to improve his learning, (2) evaluation of a learner is only part of any systematic program evaluation, (3) evaluation should occur throughout the design and implementation of a program, and (4) instructors can evaluate their own programs, although they may occasionally need consultation from experts.

Strategies

1. Use a short presentation and discussion format to present the principles of program evaluation. The following process of program evaluation should be explicated: (1) state the general evaluation problem to be addressed or decisions to be made, (2) sharpen the problem into specific questions to be answered, (3) design instruments and/or protocols to collect information, (4) collect data from the subjects, (5) analyze and interpret the data, and (6) make decisions or recommendations. It should be emphasized that a systematic evaluation can be undertaken without a staff of research assistants and complex statistics.

2. A case on which all participants can collaborate provides an excellent vehicle for learning. For example, participants can be divided in to groups of four, given a written outline of a residency program, and asked to design a protocol for a comprehensive evaluation. References should be available to answer questions as they arise. The protocol should be reported and discussed at the end of the period.

3. Based on participation in the case study, the group can develop a list of criteria for evaluation of instructional programs. The list can be used as a guide for develop-

ing protocols and conducting an evaluation of an educational program.

4. Evaluation data for either an actual or simulated evaluation project can be prepared and given to participants to analyze and to produce recommendations. Participants generally need guided experience in completing this aspect of the evaluation process.

5. A workbook can be used to facilitate design of an evaluation protocol. Workbooks are available commercially (Fink & Kosecoff, 1978), or one can easily be developed. Participants should plan their own evaluations and present them to the group for critique.

Suggested Topics

- Purpose of evaluation questions
- Personnel needed for evaluation projects
- Quantitative versus qualitative evaluation methods
- Subjects of evaluation
- Criteria and standards
- Data collection
- Data analysis, interpretation, and presentation

Competencies: 6.1 through 6.6.

Suggested Resource Material

Cronbach, L. J. (1963). Course improvement through evaluation. This paper is a classic but timeless justification and explanation of course evaluation.

Cronbach. L. J. (1982). *Designing evaluation of educational and social programs.* A rich source of insight and ideas about program evaluation.

Fink, A., & Kosecoff, J. (1978). *An evaluation primer and an evaluation primer workbook.* An excellent practical workbook with feasible exercises.

Forsythe, G. B., Sadler, J. C., & de Bliek, R. (1986). Evaluating educational programs. In W. C. McGaghie & J. J. Frey (Eds.), *Handbook for the academic physician.* An excellent brief outline and summary of the evaluation task faced by any instructor.

Whitman, N. A., & Cockayne, T. W. (1984). *Evaluating medical school courses: A user-centered handbook.* A very readable pamphlet with many useful suggestions about course evaluation.

Rationale for the Domain Design

Several issues influenced the design of courses and other strategies for the Education domain. First is the realization that not all faculty will need all aspects of the program. Preceptors generally have an isolated responsibility for education, for example. They usually serve as consultants to residents in clinics for short time periods or take advanced medical students into their practices as apprentices for longer periods. Therefore their instruction is typically limited to one learner and is clinical in nature. For this reason, they would probably need to participate only in Course 101, *Clinical Instruction*. In contrast, full-time faculty members, whether in tenure-track or non-tenure-track positions, have a much broader range of teaching responsibilities. For that reason, all full-time faculty would generally find Courses 102 to 108, in addition to Course 101, applicable to their educational responsibilities.

A second issues is the notion that any type of curricular or instructional planning must be approached systematically even if it is clinical in nature. In medical education, curriculum is usually developed and agreed upon by a department. Instruction, then, is the manner in which a curriculum is manifested by the individual instructor. Single instructors, whether they are a full-time faculty member, chair of the curriculum committee, or a part-time preceptor who attends in the clinic for only one-half day per week, do not generally plan the entire curriculum. They must, however, base their instruction on a curricular plan so that any concepts and skills taught are clearly integrated into the overall program.

A third issue is that the individual learner is ultimately the only one who can learn—curriculum and teaching do not, by themselves, magically result in learning. One strives to ensure that curriculum, instruction, and learning are consistent and complementary in order to maximize the learner's chances for successful learning. The curriculum should specify the responsibilities of the institution, the instructor, and the learner. Instruction should be based on helping learners acquire demonstrable competencies and not on covering content. It should stimulate learners to become more responsible for their own learning as they mature professionally.

Fourth, the definition of a curriculum begins with a statement of goals and then sequences those goals into an organization that makes sense. The courses are sequenced according to the way instructors generally experience their responsibilities. New instructors are initially assigned a clinically related instructional task, such as precepting. Once they accomplish this, they are assigned more complex tasks in the overall educational program. They conceptualize programs based on an understanding of how people learn, write course goals and objectives, deliver instruction, assess their learners, and evaluate their programs, in that approximate order. This model, therefore, presents courses in that sequence.

The implementation of the domain is based on a systematic process adapted from the principles of adult learning and development. This process guided the organization of each course in the domain. It is as follows:

1. The participant should perceive a specific need and application for the material presented.
2. The participant should understand and agree to the expectations for the instruction, which have been systematically planned and sequenced.
3. Information should be obtained from one or two short but specific readings prior to beginning each session.
4. A short presentation or lecturette by the leader should begin each session. Insofar as possible, it should model the strategies being taught.
5. To assist the participants in acquiring "ownership" of the concepts taught, the leaders could use group discussion to specify and achieve consensus on criteria for describing the concept being taught. This is based o n the discovery learning concept.
6. A group exercise should facilitate application of the concepts. An analysis of a written case study, a review of a videotape simulation, or examination and critique of materials can focus the application process. The topic can be an actual or simulated situation.
7. Each participant should have the opportunity to have some meaningful practice and acquire feedback, either in the structured group setting or on an individual basis. Application of the educational concept to each participant's educational responsibilities is critical. This occurs with guided practice, followed by consultation and feedback.

The Education domain maximizes these principles of systematic planning, discovery learning, group discussion, and guided practice by application. It should have an impact on a variety of medical faculty members engaged in learning new concepts and skills for use in fulfilling their daily educational responsibilities.

Annotated Bibliography

The references below were considered especially important in defining and developing this domain. Therefore, they have been annotated, while other cited works have been included only in the Reference Section. (For complete citations of these annotations and all the writings mentioned in this domain, turn to the Reference Section at the end of this chapter.)

Annotations can be very illuminating to readers for a number of reasons. First, they give readers who are not particularly familiar with the subject matter some important background information—a kind of "Cliff's Notes" to the curriculum content. Second, many of the annotations point to specific chapters or excerpts that may stimulate new ideas for teaching or provide "quick-and-dirty" teaching materials. Third, they can help direct whatever further literature searches you may be planning in the area on your own.

Last, but not least, the discerning reader will learn much about the content expert's version, or perspective, or philosophic stance regarding his or her subject by reading these deliberately selected annotations. Perhaps even more than the prose in each rationale section, this bibliography may help you to see the subject matter as the content expert saw it and to understand why the domain is structured the way it is.

Bland, C., Ullian, J., & Froberg, D. (1984). *User-centered evaluation.*

This paper discusses program evaluation from the user's perspective. User-centered evaluation focuses on ways to make internal evaluation efforts relevant and useful to those requesting the evaluation. Internal evaluation is defined as "an information-collection system about program activities and outcomes so that interested persons can *use* the information." The authors describe three characteristics of user-centered evaluation approach: (1) an ordered set of steps, (2) identification of both evaluator and decision-maker roles, and (3) careful consideration of the communication aspects of evaluation.

The steps involved in this approach are (1) identify the decision maker or primary information user for the evaluation data; (2) identify the decisions that require evaluation data and put them in order of priority; (3) determine the design, data collection strategy, and sources to be used; and (4) determine a deadline and format for reporting results.

Dinham, S. M., & Stritter, F. T. (1986). *Professional education. In M. C. Whittrock (Ed.), Third handbook of research on teaching.*

This chapter offers new faculty members an overview of the unique characteristics of the clinical component of professional educational. A definition and review of the literature on professional education are presented first, followed by a detained summary of the literature on the professional apprenticeship. Seven aspects of the apprenticeship are described: (1) prerequisite student attributes, (2) preparation for clinical education, (3) sites for apprentice learning, (4) characteristics of clinical instructors, (5) supplementary teaching strategies, (6) evaluation of student performance, and (7) evaluation of clinical teaching. The authors conclude that students' clinical performance cannot be reliably predicted; students' preparation for clinical training must include more than cognitive knowledge; and components of effective clinical teaching include attitudes and role modeling as well as organization, practice, and evaluation. They also state that content of clinical education is dictated by daily works demands; evidence of the impact of differences in clinical sites is still inconclusive; clinical performance can be reliably and validly evaluated; and teaching performance can be evaluated. Recommendations for future research in professional education are included in the final section of the chapter.

Foley, R. P. (1983). *Instructional media and methods. In C. H. McGuire, R. P. Foley, A. Gorr & R. W. Richards (Eds.), Handbook of health professions education.*

This chapter reviews the last two decades of research on instruction in health professions education. The author describes this period of research as one in which "innovative techniques were developed in response to technological advances, the proliferation of knowledge, students' increasing dissatisfaction with their education, and a general questioning of the adequacy of the health care delivery system" (p. 234). The research on instruction in health professions education includes research on instructional technology, methods, and approaches. The author offers a critical review of the studies in each of these areas, paying special attention to the adequacy of the methodologies. A summary of studies assessing student learning preferences and styles is also provided.

Most of the research on instructional technology during this period compared the effectiveness of one form of medium to another.

Studies of three types of media are discussed: Simulation, television, and self-instruction indicated an increase in student time saving and the transfer of learning from simulators to patients. Studies of television as an instructional medium show that in medicine it was as effective as lecture-demonstration, and in continuing education it was as useful as workshops. Self-instructional programs (including slide-tape, computer-assisted instruction, programmed materials, audio-tapes, and videotapes) were most often compared with conventional modes of instruction and found to be more efficient in terms of student time expended, and particularly helpful for less able students.

Studies of instructional methods also compared the effectiveness of one approach with that of another. Studies most often compared the lecture method with other approaches and showed inconclusive results. The reviewer maintains that these investigators failed to draw upon findings from studies in general education that have shown that certain methods are more effective than others in promoting particular learning outcomes.

A number of studies compared teacher- versus student-centered instructional approaches such as students teaching each other, independent study programs, and problem-based learning. Results suggest that students prefer their peers as instructors and learn as much or more from them as they do from faculty. However, research on independent study programs and problem-based learning indicated that McMaster University graduates' clinical performance in postgraduate training was equal or superior to their counterparts elsewhere.

Friedman, C. P., Slatt, L. M., Baker, R. M., Cummings, S. B. (1983). *Identifying the content of family medicine for educational purposes: An empirical approach.*

This article describes an approach to curriculum planning for medical student education. The approach includes two phases of data collection: The first determines what should be included in the curriculum, and the second assigns priorities to the content identified. Data are collected by personal interview in the first phase and questionnaires in the second. The advantages of this two-step process are that it results in a general consensus of what should be included in the curriculum and yields quantitative data concerning the relative importance of each item.

In the application presented, developers began by selecting a group of 40 individuals from all facets and levels of family medicine education at one university and from affiliated programs across the state. These individuals were interviewed and sufficient data gathered to formulate a complete description of the content of a family medicine curriculum. From these data the investigators developed a list of 27 content elements, which were organized hierarchically into four areas.

The next phase of the process began with the development of a questionnaire based on paired comparisons. Respondents were asked to choose the element in each pair that they considered more important in the education of medical students. The four areas identified in this process were (1) "Family Medicine as a Synthesis of Content and Process," (2) "Family Medicine as a Field of Inquiry," (3) "Family Medicine as a Career and Peer Group," and (4) "Family Medicine as a Value System."

As a result of this curriculum planning effort, several new departmental offerings were developed and existing offerings were revised. For the new offerings, the study results were used to develop educational goals and objectives. In addition, this information served as a planning tool to determine where high-priority areas were not being addressed by existing departmental course offerings.

Gagne, R. M., & Briggs, L. J. (1987). *Principles of instructional design (3rd ed.)*

This book gives those responsible for curriculum development a comprehensive overview of the instructional design process, from design to implementation and evaluation. The authors have developed a systematic approach to designing instruction that can be applied to any content and any educational setting.

The text is divided into four major sections. Part 1 presents a rationale for instructional design and a model of the 14 stages of instructional system design. Part 2 includes definitions and examples of the five major classes of learning outcomes: (1) intellectual skills, (2) cognitive strategies, (3) information, (4) attitudes, and (5) motor skills. In addition, the authors describe the specific conditions of learning applicable to each of these capabilities. Part 3 gives the reader a detailed procedure for designing instruction, including analyzing the learning task, writing instructional objectives, determining the instructional sequence, selecting media and methods, designing individual lessons, and assessing student performance. Part 4 addresses delivery systems for instruction and includes information on both group and individualized instruction, as well as procedures for evaluating instructional programs.

Gil, D. H., Heins, M., & Jones, P. B. (1984). *Perceptions of medical faculty members and students on clinical clerkship feedback.*

This study provides clinical instructors with information about the importance of giving feedback as a part of the instructional process. Feedback is defined as "information from instructors to learners about their past performance on the wards which serves to enhance or modify future actions of the learners" (p. 856).

The literature on feedback indicates that it is a "useful instructional technique that provides a powerful incentive to efficient learning if it is done without delay, is explicit and is clear" (p. 856). It is distinguished from evaluation in that it is aimed not at documentation, but rather at improvement of performance.

The authors conclude that the large discrepancies between faculty members' and students' perceptions of the feedback (provided or received) raise implications for future research in this area. Future studies should explore the relationship between the type of feedback provided and faculty members' training, philosophy of learning, and theories of teaching and learning. In addition, researchers should explore faculty and students' expectations about feedback with their perceptions of their respective roles. It would also be helpful to determine what constitutes an "adequate" feedback process for both students and faculty.

Guilbert J. J. (1984). *How to devise educational objectives.*

This article gives new teachers a simple yet complete explanation of what educational objectives are, what they are not, and how they are used. The introduction warns readers that educational objectives are only means to an end, and that objectives that address questionable goals are of little value. The emphasis is on how to formulate and use educational objectives in a "learning by objectives" approach.

Educational objectives can range from a very general to a most specific level, and this continuum can be divided into basic levels: (1) professional functions, (2) professional activities, and (3) professional tasks. Examples from health professions training programs are given for each level. Educational objectives can be constructed on the basis of health professionals' specific tasks. Several procedures for obtaining this data are described, including critical incident, job analysis, prospective studies, morbidity and mortality statistics, and interviews or questionnaires with health professionals.

The author concludes that the learning by objectives approach has not been widely applied in the training of health professionals. Previous misuse of this approach should not dissuade health professionals from using it. In fact, a major advantage of implementing objectives-based learning is to allow researchers to study the approach in order to improve it.

Harden, R. M. (1984). *Educational strategies in curriculum development: The SPICES model.*

This article gives new faculty members an explanation of the major curricular issues confronting educators and administrators at all medical schools. The author identifies six educational issues related to the medical school curriculum and presents each issue as a continuum between two extremes. The education strategies discussed include student-centered versus teacher-centered learning, problem-based learning versus information gathering, integrated teaching versus discipline-based teaching, community-based versus hospital-based education, elective versus a standard program, and systematic approach versus an apprenticeship. Strategies listed first are more innovative; those listed second are more traditional. While the issues are clearly interrelated, the authors present each issue separately and list factors that support a move toward innovation and those that support tradition. Newer medical schools tend to use the more innovative strategies, while established medical schools tend to use the more traditional.

The author's purpose in preparing this summary was to help readers understand curricular strategies in medical education and to give them an instrument to help with curriculum analysis, review, and development. They also address teaching methods and assessment. The author concludes that each medical school must determine where it stands on the SPICES continuum.

Irby, D. M. (1978). *Clinical teacher effectiveness in medicine.*

This study gives clinical teachers information on the specific teaching behaviors that are most and least effective in the clinical setting. The purpose of the study was to identify the characteristics of the best and worst clinical teachers as described by medical school faculty, residents, and students at the University of Washington. In addition, the responses were analyzed to determine whether the ratings were influenced by professional role, faculty department, or teaching method used.

The author identified seven important components of effective clinical teaching: (1) instructor organization, (2) relations with students, (3) enthusiasm, (4) knowledge, (5) clinical supervision, (6) clinical competence, and (7) modeling of professional standards and values. A questionnaire incorporating these components was then administered to selected faculty members, residents, and fourth-year medical students. Results showed that the best clinical teachers in the study were characterized by their enthusiasm, clarity and organization of presentation, and clinical competence. The worst teachers lacked these skills and were described as having negative personal attributes, Additional statistical analyses of the results indicated that the ratings were not unduly influenced by the professional role of the rater, department affiliation of the faculty member, or teaching method employed. In addition, the components that most effectively separated the best from the worst clinical teachers were enthusiasm, organization and clarity of presentation, and interaction skills.

Irby, D. M. (1983). *Evaluating instruction in medical education.*

This article describes a comprehensive evaluation system that integrates quantitative measures and descriptive documentation with qualitative judgments while maintaining some degree of departmental flexibility in implementation.

The evaluation system described here was designed by a faculty committee over a 3-year period. The committee's goals were to assess the current status of faculty (teaching) evaluation in the medical school and to develop a model program for evaluating instruction. Their final report included five parts: (1) purposes and university policies for evaluating teaching, (2) evaluation instruments, (3) activities for faculty members to evaluate and improve their own teaching, (4) departmental peer review of teaching procedures, and (5) specific recommendations to implement the total evaluation system.

Qualitative measures used in this system included learners' ratings of classroom instruction, clinical teaching, continuing medical education teaching, and academic advising. Qualitative judgments were made by committees overseeing peer review of teaching. These committees reviewed the qualitative measures as well as the descriptive documentation provided by the faculty member. Faculty members were responsible for maintaining a record of their responsibilities for teaching, committee assignments, course assignments, and administration.

Mattern, W., Weinholtz, D., & Friedman, C. P. (1983). *The attending physician as teacher.*

This paper describes a study investigating specific behavioral characteristics of effective clinical instruction. Six medical ward teams were randomly selected as subjects. Rounds and other activities of these ward teams were observed, and interviews with individual team members (including the attending physicians) were conducted. The information was then indexed and cross-referenced by topic. Analysis of the data revealed 11 areas in which specific actions of attending physicians appeared to contribute to instruction. These instructors: (1) allocated time for instruction both during and outside of ward rounds, (2) established a climate of trust by demonstrating concern for both patients and team members, (3) established their clinical credibility as general internists, (4) held initial orientation for ward team members, (5) conducted some type of final evaluation, (6) listened carefully to case presentations, (7) directed case discussions, (8) offered brief, relevant didactic presentations, (9) conducted bedside visits when appropriate, (10) demonstrated concern for psychosocial issues, and (11) shared teaching responsibility with other group members as necessary. The authors conclude that specific characteristics of effective clinical instruction can be identified and evaluated, and this information could be used to develop a program of systematic instructional improvement.

McGuire, C. H. (1983). *Evaluation of student and practitioner competence. In C. McGuire (Ed.), Handbook of health professions education.*

This review summarizes the last 20 years of research on the evaluation of professional competence. Innovations in professional evaluation in the late 1960s and early 1970s addressed several areas of concern: (1) the purpose of evaluation, (2) the techniques of determining essential components of competence, (3) the range of competencies assessed, (4) the methods of evaluation employed, (5) the approaches to scoring and reporting performance, and (6) the criteria used in setting standards.

Research on the purpose of evaluation indicated to the authors a new emphasis on formative evaluation, including diagnostic testing, needs assessment, student progress monitoring, and self-assessment. Research on techniques of assessing professional competence showed "an increasing systematization of the process for utilizing expert judgement and for incorporating relevant empirical sources in defining its dimensions" (p. 212).

Studies about evaluation instruments included research on traditional tests, simulation exercises, written simulations, and patient management problems (PMPs). The author concluded that the most important new development in this aspect of professional evaluation is the use of simulation and gaming theory. The section on PMPs includes a detailed discussion of validity and reliability issues, as well as a comparison of PMPs with other measures of competence. Research on computer simulations, oral simulations, and multimedia (or three-dimensional) simulators is also reviewed. A summary of the research on techniques for assessing clinical performance included both cognitive and noncognitive skills and attitudes. Research on scoring and reporting performance, as well as setting standards of adequacy, was prompted by concern to increase the validity and utility of professional evaluation and to minimize the undesirable side effects of this process. Other aspects of professional evaluation that have been investigated are competence over time and patterns of competence.

Medio, F. J., Reinhard, J. D. & Maxwell, J. A. (1984). *Improving teaching rounds: Action research in medical education.*

This study gives faculty members specific strategies for improving teaching rounds as well as a detailed description of the action research process that was used to identify and solve the teaching problems in this department. Action research is a strategy for planning and accomplishing change by involving members of the client group in the design, implementation, and evaluation of change in order to increase their ownership of the change process.

An initial diagnostic study of teaching rounds was used to collect data that would identify areas of improvement. Interviews and observations resulted in identification of five main problem areas: (1) lack of respect for teaching rounds by both attendings and house staff, (2) differing needs and knowledge levels of students, interns, and residents, (3) disagreement among attending physicians regarding bedside teaching, (4) attendings' failure to exercise adequate leadership, and (5) house staff perceptions that their evaluations of attendings were ignored.

These results were shared with faculty members who, in turn, developed an action plan. They created two committees—one to establish a set of guidelines for conducting rounds, the other to revise the form for evaluating teaching attendings.

In the follow-up study, house staff perceived a definite improvement in teaching rounds. A high percentage of attending physicians reported changes in their conduct of rounds. Specific changes were reported in four areas: (1) the setting of ground rules, expectations, and purposes of rounds, (2) scheduling and promptness, (3) fewer interruptions, and (4) bedside teaching. Continuing problems included: (1) quality of bedside teaching, (2) feedback, (3) punctuality, and (4) interruptions. The results of the follow-up study show that teaching rounds have improved in areas addressed by the printed guidelines and orientation sessions.

Neufeld, V. R., Norman, G. R. (Eds.). (1985). *Assessing clinical competence.*

This collection of essays, written by the Health Sciences faculty at McMaster University, thoroughly reviews issues involved in measuring clinical competence. While the authors present varied approaches and viewpoints, they focus on the need for a clearer definition of the full range of clinical competence, proof that it can be measured, and a positive relationship between clinical competence and the well-being of patients.

Part I describes three historical perspectives related to clinical competence; various approaches to understanding clinical competence are also explored. In Part II, criteria for evaluating methods of assessing clinical competence are reviewed. Then each of the methods are addressed in individual chapters: direct observations, oral examinations, written examinations, global rating scales, medical record review, patient management problems, computer simulations, and simulated patients. In Part III, the authors discuss the ways in which these measures can be used, especially in situations for which more than a single method is appropriate. These situations include the use of diagnostic tests, the assessment of technical proficiency, and the measurement of physician–patient interaction. In the final section, the authors synthesize the earlier sections of the book and examine future directions in four areas—education, research, certification, and health care.

Petrusa, E. R., Guckian, J. C., & Perkowski, L. C. (1984). *A multiple station objective clinical evaluation.*

This article describes a new approach to evaluating clinical performance of medical students and house staff. The authors describe the development and implementation of an Objective Structured Clinical Exam (OSCE) administered to junior medical students at the end of an internal medical clerkship. An OSCE is a series of evaluation stations where students have approximately 4 minutes to complete a very focused clinical activity. Examples include a history-taking in laboratory data, or educating a patient about a particular health condition. After performing the task, the students answer some questions about the activity. Observer/evaluators are generally used at stations where students interact with patients. In this way, as many as 30 students can rotate through 30 stations in 2 hours. The literature on OSCEs indicates that they incorporate "the same advantages as simulated and instructed patients as well as the ability to evaluate more clinical skills for more medical situations, and all in a very manageable length of time" (p. 211).

In this study a clerkship committee selected medical diagnoses that students should know by the end of their clerkship and those that were likely to have stable physical findings. The faculty were asked to identify the actual patients for the exam and to generate scripts for the history-taking cases. In addition, the patient simulators were trained, and scoring protocols were constructed. The exam included 17 activity stations and was administered to 68 students, half in a morning session and the other half in the afternoon.

The study's major finding was that student performance varied widely for any single problem and an individual student did not do consistently well or poorly on all problems. In addition, because individuals' scores varied across medical problems, it is misleading to report a single score for performance on the whole test. The authors recommend constructing a profile of performance for each student, showing levels of competence for each medical situation.

Skeff, K., Campbell, M., & Stratos, G. (1984). *Evaluation of attending physicians: Three perspectives.*

Methods of evaluating clinical teaching include ethnographic approaches, student evaluations, teacher self-evaluations, analysis of videotapes of teaching, peer evaluation, and evaluation by consultants. This study gives medical educators and administrators an evaluation design that combines several of these methods. This assessment of clinical teaching reflects the perceptions of three groups: (1) the attending physicians themselves, (2) the students and house staff, and (3) trained raters.

The subjects were 46 attending physicians from departments of pediatrics and medicine from four hospitals. To collect data on teacher opinions regarding clinical teaching, participants completed questionnaires before their teaching rotations. During the rotation, teachers were evaluated by students and house staff and by raters using videotapes of their performance. In addition, a random sample of the attending physicians completed a self-assessment.

The authors concluded that attending physicians do care about their role as clinical teachers but rate themselves low in ability in this role. In addition, attending physicians indicated only a moderate awareness of their students' and residents' opinions of their teaching performance. Moreover, both teachers and learners rated the teachers low in communication with the leaders, which indicates that teachers may need assistance with two critical parts of clinical teaching: stating expectations and evaluating learners.

Stritter, F. T., & Baker, R. M. (1982). *Resident preferences for the clinical teaching of ambulatory care.*

This study of family medicine residents' ratings of their best attending physicians gives clinical instructors information on the content areas and teaching behaviors most valued by residents. The investigators also examined the characteristics of the residents that might have influenced their decisions about what constitutes effective teaching.

Residents in six university programs were asked to identify the attending physician who they thought was the "best" clinical teacher and rate that person according to how often he addressed certain family medicine content areas and how often he demonstrated certain teaching behaviors. Then the residents were asked to respond to similar questions about a hypothetical "ideal" clinical teacher.

Results revealed that the residents felt the best clinical teachers "emphasized the use of patient management resources, primary care treatment procedures, psychosocial considerations, the business of medicine, and the knowledge of disease—in that order" (p. 38). The residents identified the most significant teaching behaviors exhibited by the best teachers as "modeling good patient care and interacting with residents." A third finding was a high degree of correlation between the residents' ratings of their best clinical teacher and their ratings of the ideal clinical teacher. The results of this study suggest that selected content areas should receive more emphasis and that the human aspects of clinical teaching may be more important than technical teaching skills.

Stritter, F. T., & Bowles, L. T. (1972). *The teacher as manager: A strategy for medical education.*

This article offers a model for improving medical education with an approach in which the teacher functions as a manager of the learning process, rather then as a resource for information. The teacher/manager creates a learning environment for the purpose of achieving predetermined objectives. The effectiveness of this approach can be evaluated easily by determining how closely the output of the system approximates its intended purpose. This method permits more time for individualized instruction and often results in more effective education.

The authors provide an example of how this approach can be used in a typical third-year clinical clerkship. The steps involved in developing this learner-oriented system include: (1) writing a statement of purpose and developing the learners' objectives, (2) developing a criterion test based on the learner objectives, (3) identifying the learning tasks, (4) designing the instructional system, (5) testing and implementing the system, (6) evaluating the learners, and (7) revising the system.

Stritter, F. T., Hain, J. D., Grimes, D. A. (1975). *Clinical teaching reexamined.*

This study gives clinical teachers specific recommendations for improving their teaching. The authors surveyed medical students to determine the specific teaching behaviors that were most helpful in facilitating their clinical learning.

The author compiled a preliminary list of clinical teaching behaviors by reviewing the literature on instructional theory and obtaining suggestions from experienced teachers. Next the list was organized into a questionnaire that was distributed to all clinical students enrolled at the University of North Carolina and the University of Alabama.

The students identified 16 specific teaching behaviors that they considered most helpful in their learning. When these items were factor-analyzed, six general teaching dimensions emerged: (1) the teacher provides a "personal environment in which the student is an active participant," (2) the teacher has a positive attitude toward teaching and students, (3) the teacher concentrates on the problem-solving process rather then factual material alone, (4) the teacher has a student-centered instructional strategy, (5) the teacher has a humanistic orientation, and (6) the teacher emphasizes references and research. The authors concluded that the most significant factor, the students' desire to be active participants in the learning process, reflects their concern about the usual teacher domination of the process. Moreover, the information from this study may be useful in developing evaluation tools and instructional materials to help clinical instructors improve their skills.

References

Abrahamson, S., & Wilkow, M. (1984). *The lecture: A problem solving unit.* Los Angeles: University of Southern California, Department of Medical Education.

Abrahamson, S., Wilkow, M., & Bartenstein, S. (1984). *The use of media.* Los Angeles: University of Southern California, Department of Medical Education.

Bandaranayake, R. C. (1986). How to plan a medical curriculum. *Medical Teacher, 7,* 7–13.

Beery, M. P. (1986). Visuals for oral and written presentations. In W. C. McGaghie & J. J. Frey (Eds.), *Handbook for the academic physician* (pp. 312–333). New York: Springer-Verlag.

Bland, C., Ullian, J., & Froberg, D. (1984). User-centered evaluation. *Evaluation and the Health Professions, 7,* 53–63.

Bonner, J. (1982). Systematic lesson design for adult learners. *Journal of Instructional Development, 6,* 34–42.

Cashin, W., & McKnight, P. C. (1985). *Improving lectures* (IDEA Paper No. 1). Manhatten, KS: Kansas State University, Center for Faculty Evaluation and Development.

Cashin, W. E., & McKnight, P. C. (1986). *Improving discussions* (IDEA Paper No. 15). Manhatten, KS: Kansas State University, Center for Faculty Evaluation and Development.

Cox, K. R., & Ewan, C. E. (1988). *The medical teacher* (chapters 4–8, 6, 10, 11, 20, 22–33). New York: Churchill-Livingstone.

Cronbach, L. J. (1963). Course improvement through evaluation. *Teacher's College Record, 64,* 672–683.

Cronbach, L. J. (1982). *Designing evaluation of educational and social programs.* San Francisco: Jossey-Bass.

Davis, R. H., Alexander, F. T., & Yelon, S. L. (1975). General principles of learning and motivation. In *Learning system design:An approach to the improvement of instruction* (pp. 198–219). New York: McGraw-Hill.

Dinham, S. M., & Stritter, F. T. (1986). Professional education. In M. C. Whittrock (Ed.), *Third handbook of research on teaching* (pp. 952–970). New York: Macmillan.

Edwards, J. C., & Marier, R. L. (Eds.). (1988). *Clinical teaching for medical residents: Roles, techniques, and programs.* New York: Springer Publishing Co.

Eichna, L. W. (1983). A medical school curriculum for the 1980s. *New England Journal of Medicine, 308*(1) 18–21.

Ende, J. (1983). Feedback in clinical medical education. *Journal of the American Medical Association, 250,* 771–781.

Fink, A., & Kosecoff, J. (1978). *An evaluation primer and an evaluation primer workbook.* Washington, DC: Capital Publications.

Foley, R. P. (1983). Instructional media and methods (pp. 234–255). In C. H. McGuire, R. P. Foley, A. Gorr, & R. W. Richards. (Eds.), *Handbook of health professions education.* San Francisco: Jossey-Bass.

Foley, R. P., & Smilansky, J. (1980). *Teaching Techniques: A handbook for health professionals.* New York: McGraw-Hill.

Forsythe, G. B., Sadler, J. C., & de Bliek, R. (1986). Evaluating educational programs. In W. C. McGaghie & J. J. Frey (Eds.), *Handbook for the academic physician* (pp. 147–169). New York: Springer-Verlag.

Friedman, C. P., Baker, R. M. (1986). An experience in curriculum development. In W. C. McGaghie & J. J. Frey (Eds.), *Handbook for the academic physician* (pp. 75–97). New York: Springer-Verlag.

Friedman, C. P., Slatt, L. M., Baker, R. M., & Cummings, S. B. (1983). Identifying the content of family medicine for educational purposes: An empirical approach. *Journal of Medical Education, 58*(1), 51–57.

Gagne, R. M., & Breggs, L. J. (1987). *Principles of instructional design* (3rd ed.). New York: Holt, Rinehart & Winston.

Gil, D. H., Heins, M., & Jones, P. B. (1984). Perceptions of medical faculty members and students on clinical clerkship feedback. *Journal of Medical Education, 59*(11), 856–864.

Guilbert, J. J. (1984). How to devise educational objectives. *Medical Education, 18,* 134–141.

Harden, R. M. (1984). Educational strategies in curriculum development: The SPICES model. *Medical Education, 18,* 284–297.

Harden, R. M., Stevenson, M., Downie, W. W., & Wilson, G. M. (1975). Assessment of clinical competence using the objective structured clinical examination. *British Medical Journal, 1*(5955), 447–451.

Heinrich, R. Molenda, M., & Russell, J. D. (1985). *Instructional media and the new technologies of instruction* (2nd ed.). New York: Wiley.

Irby, D. M. (1978). Clinical teacher effectiveness in medicine. *Journal of Medical Education, 53,* 808–815.

Irby, D. M. (1983). Evaluating instruction in medical education. *Journal of Medical Education, 58*(11), 844–849.

Irby, D. M. (1986, September, Part 2). Clinical teaching and the clinical teacher. *Journal of Medical Education, 61,* 35–46.

Kibler, R. L., Cegala, D. J., Watson, K. W., Barker, L. L., & Miles, D. T. (1981). *Objectives for instruction and evaluation* (2nd ed.). Boston: Allyn & Bacon.

Knowles, M. S. (1978). *The adult learner: A neglected species* (2nd ed.). Houston: Gulf Publishing.

Kolb, D. A. (1984). *Experiential learning*. Englewood Cliffs, NJ: Prentice Hall, Inc.

Mattern, W., Weinholtz, D., & Friedman, C. P. (1983). The attending physician as teacher. *New England Journal of Medicine, 308* 1129–1132.

McGaghie, W. (1986). Evaluation of learners (pp. 125–146). In W. M. McGaghie & J. J. Frey (Eds.), *Handbook for the academic physician*. New York: Springer-Verlag.

McGuire, C. H. (1983). Evaluation of student and practitioner competence (pp. 256–293). In C. H. McGuire, R. P. Foley, A. Gorr, & R. W. Richards. (Eds.), *Handbook of health professions education*. San Francisco: Jossey-Bass.

Medio, F. J., Reinhard, J. D., & Maxwell, J. A. (1984). Improving teaching rounds: Action research in medical education *Research in Medical Education, 23*, 283–288.

Morgan, M. K., & Irby, D. M. (Eds.). (1978). *Evaluating clinical competencies in the health professions*. St. Louis: C. V. Mosby.

Neufeld, V. R., & Norman, G. R. (Eds.). (1985). *Assessing clinical competence*. New York: Springer Publishing Co.

Olmstead, J. A. (1979). *Small group instruction: Theory and practice*. Alexandria, VA: Human Resources Research Organization.

Petrusa, E. R., Guckian, J. C., & Perkowski, L. C. (1984). A multiple station objective clinical evaluation, *Research in Medical Education, 23*, 211–214.

Popham, W. J. (1981). *Modern educational measurement*. Englewood Cliffs, NJ: Prentice-Hall.

Pratt, D., & McGill, M. (1983) Educational contracts: A basis for effective clinical teaching. *Journal of Medical Education, 58*, 462–467.

Rosenshine, B. & Stevens, R. (1986). Teaching functions (pp. 376–391). In M. C. Whittrock (Ed.), *Handbook of research on teaching*. New York: Macmillan Publishing Co.

Schwenk, T. L., & Whitman, N. (1987). *The physician as teacher*. Baltimore: Williams & Wilkins.

Skeff, K., Campbell, M., & Stratos, G. (1984). Evaluation of attending physicians: Three perspectives. *Research in Medical Education, 23*, 277–281.

Stritter, F. T., & Baker, R. M. (1982). Resident preferences for the clinical teaching of ambulatory care. *Journal of Medical Education, 57*, 32–41.

Stritter, F., Backer, R., & Shahady, E. (1986). Clinical instruction. In W. C. McGaghie & J. J. Frey (Eds.), *Handbook for the academic physician* (pp. 99–129). New York: Springer-Verlag.

Stritter, F. T., & Bowles, L. T. (1972). The teacher as manager: A strategy for medical education. *Journal of Medical Education, 47*, 93–101.

Stritter, F. T., Flair, M. (1980). *Effective clinical teaching*. Atlanta, GA: National Library of Medicine.

Stritter, F. T., Hain, J. D., & Grimes, D. A. (1975). Clinical teaching reexamined. *Journal of Medical Education, 50*, 876–882.

Stritter, F. T., & Howell, B. (1983). *A systematic approach to instruction* (35mm slide program). Chapel Hill NC: The University of North Carolina.

Weinholz, D. (1983). Directing medical student client case presentations. *Journal of Medical Education, 17,* 346–348.

Whitman, N. A., & Cockayne, T. W. (1984). *Evaluating medical school courses: A user-centered handbook.* Salt Lake City: University of Utah School of Medicine.

Whitman, N. A., & Schwenk, T. L. (1983). *A handbook for group discussion leaders: Alternatives to lecturing medical students to death.* Salt Lake City: University of Utah School of Medicine.

CHAPTER 4

Administrative Domain

Introduction to the Domain

Physician-author Lewis Thomas (1983) once wrote that "long ago, in the quiet years before World War II, being chairman of the Department of Medicine [or other specialty]... was pretty much like being head of the English department" (p. 166). Medical school departments enjoyed a fixed portion of the university's general endowment; their budgets were steady, enrollments stable, and faculty membership small. Then, with the flood of NIH dollars, a new research imperative was created. A booming health care market combined with increased numbers of students to stimulate education and patient care missions. As a result, departments "exploded." Today's academic medical centers are extremely complex, loosely organized systems. Thomas writes he would "as soon take command of a platform of scuba divers and swim into a coral reef with the notion of making improvements in its arrangement for living" as manage the "ecosystem" of a university medical school (p. 172).

Robert Friedlander (Korok, 1983) argues that the above conditions have created a "new reality" in which faculty have to "forsake academic purism" to pursue such undesirable functions as marketing, fundraising, and political activities. They have to become more accountable for their effort, income, and departmental or program mission. They have to share resources and services, consider the pragmatic benefits of research, and become clearer and more selective about what they do individually and collectively.

To function within this multifaceted environment, academic professionals need to refine their understandings of the role of academics in the health care industry and the role of health sciences in universities. Then they need to acquire knowledge in organizational development. They need to upgrade their skills in leadership, collaborative planning, conflict resolution, resource and time management, and consensus decision making. The ultimate health of academic organizations may depend upon the degree to which academic professionals acquire self-management and administrative skills.

Definition of the Administration Domain

Organizational and management development is a relatively recent field of interest whose primary literature base stems from productivity studies conducted in the 1920s and 1930s on American industry (Rothlisberger & Dickson, 1939). Interest in organizational behavior, management systems, leadership styles, and human resource development has since expanded to professional organizations. Broadly speaking, organizational development is concerned with (1) organizational health (how it can be defined and measured); (2) stages of organizational growth; and (3) organizational problems (how they can be identified and solved). The literature supporting the administration domain is concerned with the economic environment, organizational development, management, and leadership issues in professional organizations, including higher education.

Argyris (1957), Katz and Kahn (1966), Drucker (1974b), and Greiner (1972) are leading authors in organizational theory and practice. They were among the first to describe the formal and informal systems of organizations and to classify their developmental and structural processes. Additionally, Weisbord (1976, 1978) developed a model of organizational diagnosis, which he applied to academic medical centers. Zeleznik (1977), Schmidt and Tannenbaum (1960), Likert (1961), and Fisher and Ury (1983) describe the essential features of leadership and management. McCall (1982) discusses the unique demands facing leaders of professionals, and Lewis and Dahl (1976) suggest time management strategies for academicians. Gross, Gianuinta, and Berstein (1971), Giaguita (1973), Berman and McLaughlin (1973), and Havelock and Havelock (1973) provide valuable insights into the process of organizational change and the role of change agent. The environmental conflicts and constraints in academic medicine are well explained by Rogers and Blendon (1978), while Ebert and Brown (1983) review the financial trends of Academic Medical Centers of (AMCs). Academic medical center management and leadership are discussed by Strasser (1983), Delbecq and Gill (1985), and Wilson and McLaughlin (1984). Organizational and management issues, as well as problems specific to academic medicine departments, have been reported on by Aluise (1982), and Aluise, Kirkman-Liff, and Neely (1981), Aluise, Bogdewic, and Sakata (1984), and Aluise, Bogdewic, and McLaughlin (1985).

Because academic physicians perform multiple roles, they encounter three inevitable organizational dilemmas soon after beginning a faculty career. They discover that:

1. The roles of clinician, educator, and researcher often conflict, and sorting through this conflict requires special skills.
2. Academic professionals are autonomous workers who prefer to set their own objectives and define their own standards of performance; integrating them into productive work groups also calls for some special skills.
3. As individuals and as a group, faculty have to respond to external pressures to meet the needs of a diverse constituency and to compete for scarce resources.

Rationale for Including Administration in the Curriculum

One could argue that every medical center department or program could benefit from administrative development. Primary care departments may stand to gain the most, however, as they represent one of the newest specialties and are least familiar with the academic system and least experienced in organization and management in large medical centers. A more specific assessment of administrative needs in family medicine also strengthens the program or department rationale. Findings from a multisite case study analysis of academic family medicine departments indicated that organizational dilemmas previously noted are alive and well in this new discipline (Aluise, 1982). Research, teaching, and patient care priorities were seen as important, but the resources needed to achieve these missions were not well-coordinated. Although department chairs were described as innovative and energetic, they usually functioned as benevolent dictators with a centralized decision-making structure. Because performance and promotion criteria were vague, faculty found it difficult to manage their careers; there were few systematic means for integrating individual work preferences and career goals with department objectives. And, finally, many family medicine department faculty experienced conflictual relationships with faculty and administrators in other departments and the hospital.

How the Domain Has Been Structured

To distill all that physician faculty need to learn about the administrative roles and responsibilities of academic medicine professionals, the domain was divided into four areas: Environment, Organization, Leadership, and Management (see Table 4.1 below).

Environment and Organization represent the "macro" realm of administrative development. These topics deal with the issues that lay outside the immediate control of any single faculty member but tremendously influence all aspects of the academic physician's role. Environment concerns national issues in health care, medical education, and life science research, such as the trend toward alternative health systems, cost containment, the emphasis upon ambulatory care, and health promotion and disease prevention. Organization focuses on the internal structures and processes of the university, medical school, and clinical departments. Leadership and Management deal with the "micro" dimensions of academic administration—the specific tasks over which individual faculty have some control or authority. It should be clarified here that in professional organizations, leadership functions can be performed by many persons, regardless of their formal titles. Management refers to planning, organizing, and evaluating one's own work as well as the work of others.

Assumptions Made in Constructing the Domain

When people think of the word *administration*, they often think of a hierarchical governance system. The philosophical bias of our approach leans toward a more collegial form of organization and management. Academic medicine cannot fulfill its research, patient care, and teaching missions based upon autocratic methods. The management of professionals requires a balance between academic

TABLE 4.1 Subareas in the Administration Domain

Environment	*Organization*
• Economics	• Mission
• Politics	• Authority
• Constituents	• Goals/objectives
Leadership	*Management*
• Management of professionals	• Planning
• Organizational change	• Supervision
• Directing groups	• Evaluation

and corporate worlds. As McCall suggests, professionals need to be orchestrated rather than commanded by authoritarian rule.

Because of this view, we believe that all academic professionals, and particularly new faculty, need to become "students of their own organization." They need to learn about the organization that affects them and become contributing members in the management system. Too often administration is interpreted as something reserved for those in senior positions or something that gets in the way of other roles. While administrative competence is unquestionably critical for leaders, it is also critical for other members of the organization. The demands of the "new reality" of academic medical centers requires that all faculty members be empowered with administrative knowledge, skills, and attitudes.

In conclusion, knowledge of organizational and management principles and the acquisition of the corresponding skills has a twofold effect. First, they enable individual faculty members to establish a better self-management system to accomplish research, patient care, education, and administrative responsibilities. Second, they enable faculty to effectively plan, direct, and supervise projects and programs. Both dimensions are essential for academic organizations to successfully achieve their missions.

Goals and Competencies

Listed below are the goals and competencies for the Administration domain. This list represents the full spectrum of knowledge and skills required of faculty in academic medicine. It is not broken down by institution or faculty type. For suggestions on how to identify relevant competencies for preceptors, non-tenure-track, and tenure-track faculty, see Chapter 2.

These goals and competencies were prepared by the content expert after engaging in an extensive literature review, meeting with physician liaisons and advisory committee members, and reviewing the results of three surveys. The competencies are presented according to each subarea of the domain, as illustrated in Table 4.1.

Environment

GOAL 7.0: To understand how environmental pressures and trends (e.g., economic, political, societal, and organizational) affect academic medical centers.

Environment addresses the external influences that affect the health care field in general and medical education and research organizations in particular. Faculty in academic medical centers and community hospital must stay abreast of certain economic and political changes. Health care megatrends to be monitored include the increasing emphasis on consumer orientation; dominance of large-scale health organizations; emergence of prospective and prepayment plans; formation of utilization review and cost control programs by government and industry; the shift from hospital to ambulatory care; and the competition for research funding. These trends will impact medical education and research as well as health care delivery. For this reason, faculty must maintain a working knowledge of these issues to gauge the effects on their individual work and departmental programs.

Faculty should be able to:

7.1. Identify the constituencies, such as governmental agencies, industry groups, and large segments of the consumer population that their organization(s) serve
7.2. Analyze the current economic and political situation(s), research and education trends directly affecting their institution and program
7.3. Contribute to organizational planning and problem solving as it applies to economic and political issues

Organization

GOAL 8.0: To understand the formal structures of and relationships between the organizations they serve (e.g., department, medical school, university).

Whereas environment competencies focus on the external situation, organizational competencies concern the internal system. Organizational members need to understand the workings of their organization if they are to participate in or lead programs or projects successfully. Weisbord (1978) and Delbecq and Gill (1985) suggest that academic medical centers are unique organizational systems in which academic professionals must be cognizant of the competing authority structures and be prepared to negotiate when confronted with conflicting demands for resources and services.

Faculty should be able to:

8.1. Determine how their department or program goals relate to the overall mission of the institution

8.2. Describe the parallel faculty and administrative governance structures of their institution

8.3. Describe the institutional and departmental judicial process according to Delbecq's (1985) three criteria for justice: representative structure, visibility of decisions, and clarity of decision-making rules and policies

8.4. Describe the organization's decision-making process regarding finance, personnel, and program responsibilities

8.5. Identify the organization's stage of development according to Greiner's (1972) criteria of creation, direction, delegation, and consolidation

8.6. Evaluate the mechanisms that enhance an organization's strength, such as automation, performance appraisal, management expertise, planning, and evaluation process

8.7. Determine if their organization is receptive to organizational change, and facilitate the appropriate change strategy as an internal change agent

Leadership

GOAL 9.0: To participate in and provide leadership for small and large group academic tasks (e.g., direct residency program, conduct strategic planning, serve on promotions committee).

Faculty members will be called upon to serve in a variety of leadership roles. Leadership in professional organizations is perhaps one of the most demanding of all organizational roles. In McCall's (1982) report on the leadership of professionals, he concludes that professionals prefer to make their own decisions about their work priorities and use of resources. They also demand a voice in planning and decision making that has any influence upon their work. Thus, leadership of professionals is more an orchestration that a direct application of authority. McCall suggests that to lead a professional organization, a person must demonstrate a high degree of competence in the field, utilize a participative approach for planning and decision making, and respect others' needs for self-regulation.

Faculty should be able to:

9.1. Identify personal leadership styles (i.e., directing, coaching, participating, delegating)

9.2. Use a contingency model of leadership, which states that whether the leader intervenes in a highly directive or non-directive manner depends upon the maturity of the group and various situational factors

9.3. Demonstrate group leadership skills to achieve both the task and socioemotional requirements for effective group work

9.4. Identify sources of conflict (information, methods, goals, values) and apply appropriate strategies to resolve conflict

9.5. Foster a collaborative environment, characterized by respect for differences, freedom of expression, and consensus decision-making

Management

GOAL 10.0: Manage self, others, money, and time on various projects and programs.

Management is primarily concerned with resource utilization. The principal resources of an organization are people, money, and time. Regardless of the faculty member's responsibilities, managing one or more of these resources will occur very early in organizational work. First, and most important, the individual professional must establish a self-management system. Stone (1980) suggests that if academic physicians want self-direction in their professional roles they must be prepared to set priorities, integrate their objectives into the goals of the organization, establish evaluation criteria for each of their major responsibilities, and report results against a predetermined set of objectives. As faculty members assume more departmental or program responsibilities, they will need to expand their managerial skills to include budgeting, supervision, and evaluation of others.

Faculty should be able to:

10.1. Establish a self-management system similar to Stone's (1980) model that includes negotiated goals and objectives, multiple evaluation sources, and a regular review and reporting process

10.2. Hire, train, supervise, and evaluate personnel

10.3. Manage their time by prioritizing objectives, scheduling major activities, assigning and delegating tasks, and monitoring work of others

10.4. Conduct effective meetings by planning the meeting ahead

of time, using time-specific agenda items, facilitating group
discussion, using consensus decision making, and distribut-
ing written summaries

10.5. Interpret and prepare financial and other accountability reports

Courses, Strategies, and Resources

*Listed below are suggested courses, strategies, and resources for
teaching the competencies and achieving the goals of the administration
domain. Competencies to be achieved by each course or activity are listed by
number after each description. These activities and sources cover the full range
of skills identified in Administration; they are not keyed to specific faculty types
at particular institutions. For guidelines on how to select and combine courses
in this and other domains for preceptors, non-tenure-track, and tenure-track
faculty, see Chapter 8.*

*The following courses and activities will be particularly helpful to readers
who are designing administrative development programs. Individual faculty wish-
ing to attend an existing program can select one from the many nationally recognized programs mentioned later in this section. Currently, many universities,
national associations, and regional medical centers offer a variety of administrative development programs.*

201. ENVIRONMENTAL TRENDS (One full-day seminar)

Participants in this day-long seminar receive a comprehensive overview of the economic and political trends in health care and the
subsequent shifts in medical education, research, and service that
are occurring. The seminar's basic strategy is to arrange for a panel
of experts from industry, government, alternative health plans,
National Institutes of Health (NIH), the Association of American
Medical Colleges (AAMC), and academic medical centers to speak
on a range of issues. Participants submit questions in advance so
that presenters prepare for and discuss their most relevant concerns. The goal is to acquire a global sense of the environmental
context of academic medicine.

Key factors influencing the medical marketplace have been
listed below. These factors should be incorporated into the seminar program as topics.

Trends

- Wider acceptance of alternative delivery systems
- Consumer's desire for convenience, availability, and lower costs

- Extensive use of advertising and promotions
- Large health care organizations expanding into ambulatory and primary care
- Closer monitoring of hospital and physician practice patterns

Competition

- Business and government coalitions
- For-profit and nonprofit organizations
- Increasing numbers of medical and surgical specialists
- Multitude of Health Maintenance Organization (HMO) and Preferred Provider Organization (PPO) plans
- Urgent care centers and ambulatory surgery centers

Cost Containment

- Higher deductables and co-payments
- Prospective payment and standard fees
- Competitive bidding
- Incentives for outpatient care
- Self-insurance
- Utilization review and quality assurance

Competitive Strategies

- Multispecialty group practices
- Emphasis on patient education and preventive services
- Expansion of practice services—on- and and off-site
- Associations with other providers and health systems
- Ambulatory procedures and ancillary services within practice

Competencies: 7.1 through 7.3.

Suggested Resource Material

See references listed in the Annotated Bibliography under Environment. (Complete citations are listed in the Reference section) Additional materials can be obtained from organizations that publish current data on the economics of health care service, education, and research, such as the Health Care Financing Administration (Baltimore, MD); Group Health Association (Washington, DC); and the American Medical Association (Chicago, IL).

American Medical Association. (published bi-annually). *The environment of medicine; Report of the council of Long Range Planning
and Development.* Chicago: Author.
Group Health Association, 1129 20th Street, N.W., Washington, D.C.
20036. Publishes newsletter, journal, and annual reports on the
status of HMOs.
Nash, D. (1987). *Future practice alternatives in medicine.*
Sorkin, A. (1986). *Health care and the changing economic environment.*

202. ORGANIZATIONAL DIAGNOSIS (Independent project, 3 full days)

Working individually, in pairs, or in small groups, participants
schedule visits to health care organizations, government agencies, and/or other academic medical centers to study the administrative issues occurring in other settings and to determine how
other institutions and organizations address problems. Participants then apply the same process to learn about the systems,
structure, and issues of their own organizations.

The purposes of an organizational diagnosis are: (1) to
describe the cultural, political, academic, and management
environment; (2) to determine if corporate and individuals' goals
and objectives are being accomplished; and (3) to suggest strategies that will keep both the organization and its members
functioning satisfactorily in the future. A comprehensive
organizational diagnosis includes four major features: document
analysis, surveys, participant observation, and interviews.

Document Analysis

• Personnel roster, annual reports, accreditation and site
  visit reports, budget and other financial documents
• Published goal statements, historical documents, grants
• Curriculum guides, by-laws of affiliated institutions
• Faculty and staff compensation and benefit plans, promotion and tenure guidelines, list of research projects
  and faculty publication, and affiliation agreements and
  other pertinent contractual relationships

Surveys

• Attitude surveys of staff, residents, faculty, patients, and
  individuals outside the organization

Participant Observation

- Attendance at meetings, retreats, and other organizational events; observation of clinical, educational, research, and administrative functions

Interviews

Individual and small group sessions to answer the following questions:

- Are goals delineated for major functions? Is there consensus on goals?
- Is there a regular evaluation and review process?
- Which political and economic pressures impact the organization?
- How secure are resources? What are the most influential outside agencies?
- What is being done to expand the base of support?
- How are plans and decisions made? Is there an annual departmental retreat?
- How is the department organized? Who besides the chair has authority?
- Is there a middle management system? Where do administrators/supervisors fit?
- What are the major internal and external conflicts? How are they resolved?
- Do policies exist for administrative, clinical, and academic functions?
- Is there a performance appraisal system? Does it include career planning?
- How are rewards/incentives distributed?
- How effective is the current leadership? Do senior faculty perform leadership roles?
- What are the future leadership needs?
- How are automated systems utilized?
- What are the major achievements of the organization?

Strategies

The Organizational Diagnosis course is coordinated by an experienced faculty member and/or a management consultant who has conducted similar site visits. Faculty who have reviewed other programs or departments can also be helpful in planning the site visits. Organizations and institutions that are directly involved in the economic and political situations similar to those of the home organization should be visited. Prior to the site visits, individuals should review appropriate information about the organization, schedule meetings with key individuals, and read articles and publications relevant to the topics. The diagnosis should include: (1) review of goals and objectives, (2) assessment of the external influences, (3) analysis of organizational authority and decision making, (4) identification of major conflicts and how they are resolved, (5) determination of leadership styles and their effectiveness, and (6) mechanisms in place that assist the organization and its members in achieving corporate and individual goals.

Possible organizations to visit are the Health Care Financing Administration, health care coalitions, health maintenance organizations, and insurance companies. In addition to these institutions, academic physicians can also visit other academic medical centers and/or community hospitals. Such investigation should again focus upon organizational, leadership, and management issues, particularly those that are relevant to health care and medical education.

The course concludes with written report prepared as a case study analysis. Qualitative research guidelines will apply, which include document analysis, participant observer reports, interview summaries, and opinion surveys. Each case study investigation will be reviewed with the advisor and peers midway through the diagnosis, and then a final presentation will be made at the end of the program.

Competencies: 8.1 through 8.7.

Suggested Resource Material

See the references in the Annotated Bibliography under Organization. Weisbord's text *Organizational Diagnosis* (1978) provides the basic concepts and should be used as the learner's text to guide the investigation and analysis of the project. Mintzberg's book *The Structuring of Organizations* (1979) presents an excellent description of the unique features of various organizational systems, including professional bureaucracies such as academic medical centers. Aluise (1982) applied Weisbord's organizational diagnosis model to the structure and function of Family Medicine departments. Complete citations are in the Reference section.

203. STRATEGIC PLANNING WORKSHOP (Two 3-hour sessions)

After participating in 201 (Environmental Trends Seminar) and 202 (Organizational Diagnosis), participants are ready for a strategic planning workshop. This two-part workshop focuses first on the impact of specific economic, political, and other trends on their immediate organization, and second on the strategic planning process. Cope's (1978) guidelines suggest the 10 steps necessary for strategic planning in an academic organization:

1. Examine existing statements of purpose. A statement of purpose or philosophy provides a foundation for direction.
2. Engage in discussion of the future and formulate a list of assumptions. Identify shifting values, new skills, constraints, and other future issues the strategy must address.
3. Describe the organization (or subunit) and its service area or commitment. List teaching, research, patient care, and other major elements that the plan must accommodate. Who are the constituencies? What are the unique features? What outcomes are possible?
4. Identify major strengths. List assets, both human and material. Indicate favorable relations and past successes that have value in the future.
5. Identify major weaknesses. List liabilities or deficiencies. Indicate the major challenges or barriers that must be overcome. State the "unresolvable" issues that must either be tolerated or circumvented.
6. Reidentify the assumptions, particularly about the future. Indicate the potential positive/negative impact. Submit minority report if a few have strong feelings about future issues.
7. Make a new statement about mission and goals. Describe where you would like to go. Specify new outcomes and how these are the same or different from past goals and results.
8. Determine guiding objectives (means, milestones). Objectives provide a guide to decision making. They also aid in working out details and assigning responsibilities.

9. Make additional modifications to missions, goals, and objectives. Distinguish between the "ideal" and the "realistic" possibilities. Specify the 1-year, 2-year, and 5-year feasibility of accomplishing goals and objectives.
10. Synthesize all that is known and design strategic alternatives. The planning group must ultimately identify and emphasize programs and resources; assign responsibility; specify action(s); obtain necessary approval; and set dates for monitoring and evaluating results.

Strategies

Arrange for one or two speakers to present on strategic planning processes and to illustrate how this organizational tool can be applied to problems occurring in academic medical centers. Participants practice planning in small groups, using Cope's (1978) model and information from advance readings. A suggested agenda might include:

- presentation recapping major problems and environmental trends in health care
- presentation of strategic planning process models
- small group discussion
- feedback to presenters from small groups
- strategic plans developed by participant groups
- review of plans and critique by presenters and other participants

Competencies: 7.1 through 7.3.

Suggested Resource Material

See references in the Annotated Bibliography under Environment. For further suggested materials the Reference section contains complete citations. The AMA also publishes a bi-annual report entitled the *Environment of Medicine* that can be used as a reading assignment before the workshop. Additional sources are:

Cope, R. G. (1978). *Strategic policy planning. Project planning exercise.* Human Synergistics. Plymouth, MI.
Lorange, P., & Vancil, R. F. (1976, September–October). How to design a strategic planning system.

204. LEADERSHIP AND MANAGEMENT SKILLS PROGRAM (16 half-day sessions)

A course of study and skill-building in organization, leadership, and management can be conducted on-site with faculty from the same department or off-site with faculty from different institutions. The content of the leadership and management skills program should be related to situations facing academic professionals.

Suggested Topics

1. *Academic Professionals:* description of the characteristics and unique features of the different roles that academic physicians must perform, i.e., patient care, education, administration, and research, and the dichotomy between organizational goals and objectives and the professionals' values and individualistic orientation.
2. *Organization Role Stress:* analysis of ambiguity, conflict, and overload in each faculty member's role; determination of the sources of stress; development of stress management strategies.
3. *Time Management:* personal and professional objectives and priorities; identification of time wasters and time savers; time allocations for the four major roles (patient care, teaching, research, and administration); time management plan that includes self-management, qualitative dimensions, and organizational requirements.
4. *Role Analysis and Negotiation:* written role description including major responsibilities, strengths, areas for improvement, and satisfaction; presentation of negotiation concepts and strategies; role play of a negotiation between faculty member and superior.
5. *Performance Appraisal:* design of an individual performance appraisal system, including role description and evaluation criteria for each of the four major roles and the process of formative and summative reviews.
6. *Leadership Styles:* analysis of personal leadership styles; feedback on behavioral types (Myers-Briggs Type Indicator); discussion of contingency leadership theory; vignettes of leadership situations.
7. *Management of Professionals:* discussion of the unique traits of professionals and the qualities needed to lead

fellow professionals; analysis of the difference between leaders and managers; review of *In Search of Excellence* (Peters & Waterman, 1982) and *Managing Professionals in Research and Development* (Miller, 1986) as they apply to academic medical organizations.

8. *Group Decision Making and Leadership of Committees:* nominal group process, force-field analysis, consensus decision making, functional and dysfunctional roles in meetings, role play and critique of a departmental meeting.

9. *Organizational Change and the Role of the Change Agent:* dealing with levels of change, knowledge, attitude, behavior, and group; change cycles (participative vs. coerced); change through behavior modification; change agent roles (Catalyst, Solution-Giver, Process Helper, and Resource Linker).

Each session should be preceded by readings or case studies. The sessions can include brief lectures, self-assessment exercises, case studies, simulations, or discussion groups. Speakers should be selected for their expertise in the content area and their ability to apply the subject to the level of academic professionals. Participants should be provided opportunities to apply the concepts to their own situation.

Competencies: 8.1 through 8.6, 9.1 through 9.5, and 10.1 through 10.5.

Suggested Resource Material

See references in the Organization, Leadership, and Management sections of the Annotated Bibliography for more materials. The Reference section contains complete citations. Other sources that provide both theory and practical examples are:

Journals that contain management education articles relevant to health care and academic medicine, such as *Health Care Management Review, Harvard Business Review, Journal of Health Care Training and Development,* and the *Journal of Training and Development.*

McGaghie, W., & Frey, J. J. (Eds.), (1986). *Handbook for academic physicians.*

Miller, D. (1986). *Managing professionals in research and development.*

Pfeiffer, J., & Jones, J. (Eds.). (published yearly.) *Handbook for group facilitators.*

205. PROFESSIONAL DEVELOPMENT PLAN (Independent project, 3 half-days)

Application of self-management concepts can best be achieved by having each faculty member develop an individual professional development plan. The professional development plan can be incorporated into the leadership and management skills program or be conducted as an independent project. An advisor should be available to assist each faculty member. As adapted from the work of Stone (1980), the fundamentals of self-management used in this project are:

1. Visibility of departmental and individual objectives
2. Setting mutually agreed-upon objectives
3. Visibility for specific roles and activities
4. Clarifying the roles to perform and desired expectations
5. Evaluation based upon predetermined, measurable objectives
6. Evaluation collected from several sources over time
7. Reporting results and willingness to negotiate changes

The professional development plan is an important mechanism for integrating the professional's values and needs into the academic medical organization. A successful professional development plan requires:

- A series of planning and feedback sessions
- Evaluation based upon specific, stated expectations
- Periodic recognition of achievements
- Mutual understanding of the areas for improvement
- Peer review to evaluate professional competence

The professional development plan should be reviewed midway through the program and then presented at the end of the program. Participants will be encouraged to design the plan based upon their individual goals and the organizational context. This plan should include a summary of their major roles and responsibilities, annual performance review guidelines, evaluation methods to be used to obtain feedback on each role, and career development needs. The plan should be reviewed with the faculty member's superior. At the final presentation, the plan should be submitted in written report form.

Competencies: 10.1 through 10.5.

Suggested Resource Material

Stone, H. (198). *Self-management: A model for professional accountability in education.*

Additional Resources

If local resources are not available to implement the courses and activities listed above, assistance can be obtained from nationally recognized administrative medicine programs, such as:

1. Group Health Association, 624 Ninth Street, N.W., Washington, DC. 20036. Conducts seminars and workshops throughout the country on health care finance topics. Their orientation is on HMOs and the economic and political issues facing prepayment plans.
2. The Physician Executive Management Center, 2901 W. Busch Blvd., Suite 600, Tampa, Florida. 33609-2517. This organization coordinates programs for the Menninger Foundation, the Association of Medical Directors, and other organizations that provide management education for physicians with administrative responsibilities. Programs are conducted nationally and range in length from 2 days to 1 week.
3. Johns Hopkins University Center for Health Care Management, 624 North Broadway, Baltimore, Maryland. 21215. A variety of educational programs (fellowships, degree programs, and workshops) are available annually.
4. University of Wisconsin Administrative Medicine Program, 1226 Observatory Drive, Madison, Wisconsin. 53706. A 3-week summer institute is conducted for physicians in leadership roles. The program also offers other on-campus courses and tutorials.
5. Department of Institutional Development, Association of American Medical Colleges, One Dupont Circle, N.W., Suite 200, Washington DC. 20036. Programs are conducted throughout the country for physicians who have major administrative roles in academic medial centers.
6. Harvard University, School of Public Health, Executive Programs in Health Policy, Cambridge, Massachusetts.

02115. A variety of programs are available, including degree programs, summer institutes, workshops, and seminars.

7. New York University, Graduate School of Public Administration, Advanced Management Program for Clinicians, 738 Tisch Hall, 40 West 4th Street, New York, New York. 10003. Offers institutes and degree programs in Health Policy and Management.

This list is not meant to be all-inclusive; leadership and management training programs for professionals are offered by most colleges, universities, industrial and government organizations, professional organizations, and specialized training organizations. Faculty development programs may have the opportunity to affiliate with local educational institutions and organizations, or faculty members can enroll as individual participants.

Annotated Bibliography

The references below were considered especially important to the content expert in defining and developing this domain. Therefore, they have been annotated, whereas other cited works have been included only in the Reference Section. (For complete citations of these annotations' and all other writings mentioned in this domain, turn to the Reference section at the end of this chapter.)

Annotations can be very illuminating to readers for a number of reasons. First, they give readers who are not particularly familiar with the subject matter some important background information—a kind of "Cliff's Notes" to the curriculum content. Second, many of the annotations point to specific chapters or excerpts that may stimulate new ideas for teaching or provide you with "quick-and-dirty" teaching materials. Third they can help direct whatever further literature searches you may be planning in the area on your own.

Last but not least, the discerning reader will learn much about the content expert's vision, perspective, or philosophic stance regarding his or her subject by reading these deliberately selected annotations. Perhaps even more than the prose in each rational section, this bibliography may help you to see the subject matter as the content expert saw it and to understand why the domain is structured the way it is.

Environment

Ebert, R. H., & Brown, S. S. (1985). *Academic health centers.*

Growth of the medical school establishment since World War II can be attributed to federal funding, increases in contributions from the medical school or university activities, state and local government, and endowments and gifts. The biggest shift in funding has been the decrease in federal funding since 1965–1966 and a subsequent increase in the proportion of funds coming from medical school activities, especially medical practice plans on a fee-for-service basis.

Academic health centers are becoming quite fragile because of the associated high costs of patient care, reductions in federal funding, and uneven distribution of federal support for research. The future of academic health centers is largely dependent on effective institutional planning, as well as departmental and divisional planning. Each academic health center will have to exploit its special strengths, seek to share teaching costs with other hospitals, and set up multispecialty group practices. Successful teaching hospitals must perform all three functions—teaching, patient care, and research—well. The AMCs must plan on an institutional basis for each of the three functions and create a reward system that recognizes the importance of each function.

This article is an excellent overview of the evolution of academic health centers. Primary care was not a part of the early and middle stages of academic health center growth; therefore, faculty can gain valuable information regarding historical trends in government support of clinical practices and research development. In addition, faculty can use the information to determine how their departmental and individual programs accomplish the three-pronged mission of patient care, teaching, and research, recognizing the constraints facing academic health centers.

Roger, D. E., & Blendon, R. J. (1978). *The academic medical center: A stressed American institution.*

The stresses that create problems for AMCs include: (1) the major role teaching hospitals serve in delivering medical care to the community, (2) the location of many AMCs in large cities, which affects the characteristics of the patient population, (3) the increased size of these medical centers, creating problems with management and governance that were previously nonexistent, and (4) the additional responsibilities given to the AMS's to correct imbalances in the distribution of medical care. Other problems are created by the AMCs' tendency to train specialists and subspecialists rather than training primary care physicians, and an increasing number of patients coming to the AMC for medical treatment of social problems such as alcoholism and marital problems.

The confrontational situation between the AMC and the federal government is detrimental to both parties and to society in general. Therefore, a mutually supportive relationship must be reestablished. The authors suggest that, first, AMCs develop cooperative linkages with other institutions, and, second, AMCs and the government agree on the number and kinds of health professionals needed and adjust training opportunities accordingly. Third, government and society must develop and support other institutions to provide "human support services," and, fourth, government and private medicine must determine the best way to provide quality medical care to all segments of the population. Fifth, all parties involved in the medical care enterprise must work together to find a solution to the cost control issue.

Discussion of the complexity of academic medicine and the problems it deals with provides academic physicians with a "real world" perspective of the field in which they have chosen to work. The authors offer many excellent suggestions to address the stresses facing medical centers, and most of their comments can be applied to primary care. This article also sheds light on the need for the various "independent" academic units to form together so that more effective strategies can be developed to deal with such pressures as cost containment, distribution of physicians, and efficient administrative structures.

Self, T. (1980). *The institutionalization of family medicine education.*

This volume provides an analysis of the impact of professional, educational, and administrative characteristics of medical schools upon the institution. Results of this study of the institutionalization of family medicine education in the United States reveal the 91% of the 126 U. S. schools of medicine have some type of family medicine unit and that 82% of the 114 family medicine units have achieved departmental status. Funding for these units is comparable to that of similar disciplines, but a substantial part of that funding is supplied by the federal government.

Measures of faculty parity revealed that the faculty are as well paid as those in other departments; however, the amount of revenue generated through their patient fees was "not very great." The average family medicine faculty member is equal in academic rank or lower than faculty in comparable disciplines, and tenure rates are lower.

Other measures of institutionalization include family medicine course requirements for undergraduates and information about family medicine residency requirements.

Results of the study show that family medicine education does not meet the "prerequisites" for traditional institutionalization. Limitations include the inability to generate sufficient practice income and inability to gain academic credibility by conducting research and publishing articles. The results indicated that rural public medical schools with state-mandated units of family medicine showed a greater degree of institutionalization than others, particularly when the residency programs were tailored to identified needs of the population.

This study provides an objective assessment of family medicine's initial development as an academic discipline. Faculty will gain an understanding of how family medicine compares to other clinical fields in such areas as sources of funding, size and caliber of faculty, and breadth of programs. This comprehensive analysis will enable faculty to appreciate family medicine's challenge as a new specialty and to compare their home department with a national profile of all family medicine departments and other clinical departments in academic medicine.

Weisbord, M., Lawrence, P., & Charns, M. (1978). *Three dilemmas of the academic medical centers.*

The authors report the results of their "action research" in nine academic medical centers over a 6-year period. Their major focus was to see whether systematic application of contingency theory to the organization and management of each academic medical center would help identify central problems relevant to AMCs. The results of the study indicate three important dilemmas facing AMCs: (1) differentiation of professional tasks, (2) integration or conflict management, and (3) local response to environmental pressures.

The data gathered on the differentiation dilemma suggest that task conflict between research, education, patient care, and administration is more of an organizational problem than an individual one. It is experienced most by administrators. Individuals manage their task conflict to their satisfaction, but experience the conflict as one with administrators rather than as inherent in the nature of their work. Managers felt that this dilemma adversely affects the institution's performance.

The integration dilemma occurs when professional autonomy, nonconfrontational management, and relatively low influence of top managers make it difficult to achieve integration either among tasks or between departments. Better coordination would require wider acceptance of confrontation, professional acceptance of legitimate authority, higher credibility for integrative tasks of management, and better definitions and measures of what constitutes good institutional performance.

Organization

Aluise, J., Bogdewic, S., & Sakata, R. (1984). *Organizational diagnosis for academic family medicine.*

This article presents a case study analysis of 10 departments of family medicine. The research questions were: How are departments organized? What are the critical organizational issues that affect family medicine's ability to develop as a discipline? What strategies will secure family medicine's position in academia? Weisbord's model of organizational diagnosis was used to analyze each department. Interviews, documents, and observations were used to collect data during a 2-day site visit.

The results of the multidepartment investigation indicated that despite the rapid growth in family medicine programs, there were many issues identified that could influence future progress. Continuing federal support is uncertain. Clinical income will need to become a larger portion of revenue. Administrative policies are loosely applied, and management systems lack sophistication. Centralized control is the norm, despite the growing size and diversity of the departments.

Conclusions from this study pointed to the need for more innovation within and outside the department, the need for training faculty for academic and managerial roles, and the need for improving the departments' financial and personnel systems.

Academic family physicians should find this study very enlightening. Perhaps they will see reflections of their own departments in the findings and conclusions. It is hoped that some of the issues that are considered problems will be recognized at an early stage and resolved. However, this study does demonstrate the need for organizational assessment and the realization that goals and aspirations in family medicine may not be achieved if the organization does not function systematically.

Drucker, P. F. (1974b). *New templates for today's organizations.*

Drucker explains that companies are suffering from organizational structures that are increasingly short-lived and unstable. The crisis is one of organization theory and organization practice. The main causes of instability are changes in the objective task, which have generated new design principles that no longer fit traditional organization concepts.

He describes the five models of organizational structure, including Fayol's functional structure, Sloan's federal decentralization, and three new ones: team organization, simulated decentralization, and systems structure. Each of these structures incorporates a logic that makes it the appropriate one to use when a particular task of management requires a structure. The dimensions of management that support these models include: (1) work and task functions, (2) results and performance functions, (3) relationship functions, and (4) decision functions. In the ideal case, an organization should be structured around all four of these dimensions. It is necessary, of course, to choose among different facets and to combine these dimensions.

The major task for management, then, is to structure the organization to satisfy the need for clarity, economy, direction of vision, understanding of tasks, decision making, stability and adaptability, and perpetuation and self-renewal. No one design principle can satisfy all of these specifications.

Drucker concludes that good organization design and structure do not just evolve; they require thinking, analysis, and a systematic approach. He also sees key tasks as "the building blocks," that must be identified and organized first. Drucker believes that organizations are not mechanical but organic and unique to each business or institution and that their structure is still merely a means for attaining institutional objectives and goals. Today's complex organizations require new designs to function effectively as well as serve "the higher goals of human endeavor."

Drucker's article is an excellent overview of organizational structures, as well as a prescription for today's academic medical center institutions. Primary care disciplines will apply many of the principles offered to establish an effective organizational system. Regardless of a faculty member's position in the department hierarchy, consideration of these concepts may be inspirational.

Greiner, L. E. (1972). *Evolution and revolution as organizations grow.*

Greiner maintains that organizational structure and process affect future growth. Growing organizations move through five phases of development, each of which contains a relatively calm period of growth or an evolution that ends with a management crisis or period of revolution.

The five influences upon organizational development include: (1) age of organization, (2) size of organization, (3) stages of evolution, (4) stages of revolution, and (5) growth rate of the industry or field. The characteristics of Phase 1 ("creative evolution") include management activities centered around making and selling a new product. The crisis for this phase is one of leadership—as the organization grows, managerial problems increase. The solution is to install a strong business manager. In Phase 2 a crisis develops from demand for greater autonomy on the part of midlevel managers. A frequent solution is to move toward greater delegation. In Phase 3 growth occurs after the successful application of a decentralized organizational structure. The crisis occurs when top executives lose control over diversified field operations. Phase 4 is characterized by top executives initiating the use of formal systems to achieve greater coordination. The red-tape crisis occurs in Phase 4 as "procedures become more important than problem solving and innovation." Phase 5 is characterized by a more flexible and behavioral approach to management. The crisis for this phase is not clear; however, it will likely be psychological burnout of employees who have been intensely involved in teamwork and searching for innovative solutions to the problems of the organization.

The author recommends that top managers identify the development stage(s) their organization is in, then recognize the specific solutions necessary for the particular phase. Then, rather than resting on their laurels, managers have to realize that solutions create problems and learn to anticipate those future problems.

This article will help faculty to understand the concept of organizational growth and to identify their department's current stage of development. Regardless of the stage their department is in, the important questions remain: What types of leadership and "followship" are needed? Is a crisis imminent? How can progress be maintained to continue growth? Faculty may use this article to become effective change agents in their home departments and perhaps assist their departments in becoming more integrated with their medical center institution.

McCall, M. W., Jr. (1982). *Leadership and the professional.*

The author looks at research on the management of professionals. He first defines professionals as individuals in occupations with prolonged specialized training, autonomy and commitment to their work, identification with the profession, a sense of ethics about professional activities, and collegial responsibility for maintenance of standards in the profession.

Research suggests that "the potential for conflict between professionals and bureaucratic organizations employing them is high;" thus, leadership presents a challenge for the managers or supervisors of these individuals. Interestingly, the author considers whether leadership of such autonomous professionals makes a difference in their performance. The research indicates that four leadership factors seem to affect professionals' productivity: (1) the supervisor's technical competence, (2) creation of a climate of controlled freedom in which decision making is shared, (3) leaders who act as a metronome, "rearranging priorities, changing sequences and responding to the ebb and flow of events," and (4) the supervisor's ability to provide challenging work.

The author continues by explaining "breakpoint leadership," which refers to the leader's ability to influence across organizational lines. The skills necessary for this type of leadership are different from those required for the supervision of a group of professionals. The final segment investigates the factors influencing a young professional's decision to pursue a career in research or management.

This monograph describes the characteristics of professionals in organizations and the challenge of managing them. Faculty in academic medicine face all the issues described in this report. They should find the information extremely helpful, especially as they assume managerial responsibilities. Faculty will need to apply the factors of professional leadership and "breakpoint leadership" if they are to succeed in directing and motivating their peers.

Weisbord, M. R. (1978). *Organizational diagnosis: A workbook of theory and practice.*

The first part of this book is a workbook on organizational diagnosis. The author presents a six-step model for understanding organizations and carefully explains the concepts and vocabulary necessary for each step. The process includes identifying the organization's purposes, its structure, its leadership, the rewards, help mechanisms, and relationships existing in the system. Worksheets accompany each step so that readers can apply the process to their particular organizational setting. The workbook is designed to help the reader to identify strong and weak points of a particular organization; identify ways to improve things in a systematic way; become aware of one's biases and assumptions; and develop a more systematic way of managing organized work.

The second half of the book consists of resource readings on each of the major concepts identified in the model, such as action research and organizational development, systems approach, informal system, purpose and mission, human side of the matrix, designing organizations to match tomorrow, management of differences, diagnosing conflict between groups in organizations, leadership, and organizational development in medical centers.

Faculty will find this book a valuable guide for understanding how their department and medical school operate as formal systems through politics and authority and as "informal" systems of relationships and interactions. By applying Weisbord's model, academic physicians can become aware of the gaps existing between the organization's intended purpose and its actual performance. This book can be an invaluable reference for faculty who are evaluating other organizations as consultants or who are interviewing for new positions. This book has also been used successfully in faculty development fellowship programs. Following a brief orientation, fellows are able to grasp the concepts and then conduct a mini diagnostic assessment of their home department.

Leadership

Delbecq, A. L., & Gill, S. L. (1985). *Justice as a prelude to teamwork in medical centers.*

Efforts to achieve teamwork and collaboration in hospitals and medical centers have been largely ineffective because the conventional rationales for team building are "unlikely motivators" in health care settings. These authors propose the use of structured decision processes to achieve cohesive problem solving and organizational justice.

Data collected on physician leaders attending the Physician-in-Management seminars indicate that they prefer not to work jointly with other professionals and have a high need for power and control. They are described as "non-collegial" and primitive "battlers" in times of conflict. However, 84% stated that they do not value authoritarianism. In addition, these "non-teamwork" behaviors tend to increase with the physician's age.

Another barrier to teamwork is the fact that medical organizations are "loosely coupled systems" in which the physicians see themselves as affiliated with, but not employees of, the organization. Moreover, physicians are willing to allot only a limited amount of time to managerial and organizational decision-making process.

For these reasons, due process becomes more effective than cohesion for strategic decision making at the macro level (between medical units or for the medical center as a whole). Physicians as a group do express a strong value toward due process, believe in majority rule, and are concerned about high morale. These values suggest that leadership in this context must include clear representative structures, visible processing of decisions, and clear decision rules.

This article is an excellent description of the difficulties physicians face as organizational members. It will be particularly beneficial for academic physicians who moved from a solo, independent orientation to the perplexing world of a medical center. Academic physicians should heed Delbecq's advice regarding the conflicting values that underlie a professional medical organization. As academic primary care programs continue to grow in size and complexity, the need for a judicial system will become more apparent. Faculty should be prepared for the enactment of procedures that will result in representation, visibility, and clarity of the "corporate" decision-making process.

Likert, R. (1961). *New patterns of management.*

This book is a classic text in management process. The author describes the properties and performance characteristics of highly effective groups. Effective groups tend to have members skilled in leadership and membership roles; members who have confidence or trust in each other and the leader; members who are willing to achieve common objectives; a group of people who are eager to assist each member to develop to his or her fullest; goals that are adapted to each member's capacity to perform; group members who communicate openly so that information is relevant and of value; and members who are eager to influence and willing to be influenced.

The author also defines leadership functions for highly effective groups. Specific leader traits include: listening well and patiently; accepting some of the blame for mistakes; allowing members the opportunity to express themselves; being careful not to impose a decision upon the group; and arranging for others to perform leadership functions.

Even though Likert's views represent the ideal, the literature on management of professionals supports many of these principles. Faculty will find that the group process and leadership guidelines suggested are useful when they are working in groups or as they prepare to take a leadership role with colleagues. If they can incorporate some of Likert's precepts, then primary care departments may evolve into more cohesive and participative units.

Prince, G. (1982). *Creative meetings through power sharing.*

Although this article concerns meetings conducted by managers with their subordinates, the author offers a wide range of ideas and suggestions to those who will lead and participate in groups. He emphasizes collaboration, cooperation, and encouragement as watchwords for effective group work, and describes the necessary approach to build a climate of approval.

Another important contribution of the article is the contrasting assumptions of a judgmental and judicious manager. The judgmental manager protects his power, describes every course of action, renews and control others, takes credit for results of groups, defines the mission, and spots flaws and applies corrective action. The judicious manager uses others to maximize group talents, shares power, recognizes accomplishments of others, gets results by helping others overcome flaws, facilitates discovery of the mission by others, and joins with others to obtain success.

This article provides more information about working effectively with others than it does on conducting meetings. The concept of "judicious manager" is important for academic physicians, whether they are working with a peer group or managing staff personnel. The success of professionals is often determined by their ability to work with others in joint ventures or to catalyze a group effort to accomplish projects or ad hoc activities. Employing the principles of a judicious manager should enhance achievement of group work.

Schmidt, W., & Tannenbaum, R. (1960). *Management of differences.*

The thesis offered in this article is that the ability to deal effectively with differences depends on diagnosing and understanding differences; being aware of and selecting appropriate behaviors; and being similarly aware of and dealing with one's feelings.

Factors that cause conflict are: (1) disagreements over facts because individuals have different information or perceptions of the information and/or position; (2) disagreement about what goals should be accomplished as definitive objectives; (3) differences about methods, procedures, strategies, or tactics; and (4) disagreement over values, ethics, moral considerations, or assumptions about such issues as equity and justice.

Choosing the appropriate conflict management approach requires answering questions such as: What is the nature of the difference? What factors influence this difference? To what stage has the interpersonal difference evolved?

Since conflict is inherent in academic medical organizations, this article is particularly valuable to academic physicians who will experience both intra- and interdepartmental conflicts, as well as interpersonal disputes among colleagues. Understanding how to diagnose conflicts and then choose an appropriate strategy will be a valuable contribution to organizational and individual productivity. In Weisbord's (1976) study of academic physicians, the most frequent method of conflict management was "avoiding" or "smoothing over." This article provides professionals an approach for confronting conflict more appropriately.

Strasser, S. (1983). *The effective application of contingency theory in health settings: Problems and recommended solutions.*

This author maintains that while contingency theory is useful in helping managers take into account differences among individual employees and situational variables, implementing contingency theory can bring about a number of problems. A realistic appraisal of its strengths and weaknesses is therefore important for critical application of contingency theory.

The contingency theory of management centers around the manager's ability to correctly identify situational determinants and then to apply strategies effectively for that particular situation. Strengths of this managerial perspective include: (1) recognition of the range of individual differences that exist among employees in complex organizations (such as health organizations), (2) recognition of the multitude of situational variables that exist in health care organizations, (3) recognition that one of several managerial responses may be needed, and (4) availability of prescriptive models that have been derived from it.

There are, nevertheless, a number of problems that arise when managers attempt to apply contingency theory. First, subordinates may perceive the manager as inconsistent. Second, managers may be forced into roles in which they are not comfortable. Time constraints and availability of quality information are additional obstacles. Moreover, subordinates may feel that their boss is operating inequitably.

The author presents several hypothetical examples in health care organizations to demonstrate these difficulties and then offers some solutions to improve the application of contingency theory. Managers can overcome these problems first by explaining to subordinates the supervisor's managerial approach. Second, they can use several different strategies to cope with the discomfort of changing supervisory styles, and, third, they can integrate their own managerial experience into the contingency theory.

Since primary care faculty will lead in a variety of situations and direct a diverse group of people, it is imperative that they understand the contingency theory of leadership. Self-assessment of leadership style and situational diagnosis are essential to applying contingency theory. As faculty become more astute in analyzing organizational situations and determining the appropriate leadership approach, they will find that administrative responsibilities may be more manageable and considerably less time-consuming.

Wilson, M. P., & McLaughlin, C. (1984). *Leadership and management in academic medicine.*

The authors' interest in the study reported here on leadership and management in academic medicine grew out of their work with the Department of Institutional Development at the Association of American Medical Colleges (AAMC). The book provides a wealth of information on environmental forces, public policy, and societal trends at medical schools. Attention is also given to the leadership and decision-making process of academic medical centers, especially at the level of dean and department head. Managerial functions, such as strategic planning, control systems, financial management, information management, and human resource management, are discussed in depth.

This book provides academic faculty with an encyclopedia of information about the characteristics, functions, and administration roles that represent the academic medical center. It should be required reading for any new member of an academic medical center department and will remain a valuable reference when faculty take on administrative responsibilities. The authors have also provided several suggested readings and "self-study."

Zaleznik, A. (1977). *Managers and leaders: Are they different?*

Every organization needs both managers to maintain operations and leaders to create new approaches and to discover new areas to explore. The author maintains that while both managers and leaders are needed, they have distinctly different world views and develop differently because each is a psychologically different type.

Managers are problem solvers and adopt impersonal attitudes toward goals, while leaders adopt an active and personal attitude toward goals. Managers tend to view work as a process that depends upon the interaction and cooperation of groups of people as they generate strategies and make decisions. They strive to limit choices, while leaders try to develop new approaches to longstanding problems. They must create excitement in work.

In addition, managers prefer to work with people and to maintain a low level of emotional development in those relationships. Leaders relate to others in more intuitive and empathetic ways and attract strong feelings of love and hate.

The author suggests that managers develop through socialization while leaders develop through personal mastery. He then gives two examples (Dwight Eisenhower and Andrew Carnegie) of how a leader's development is often dependent on a mentor relationship at some important point in his or her career.

This article presents a thought-provoking distinction between leadership and management. Academic physicians can reflect on into which camp they might tend to fall. Regardless of one's primary orientation or role, it will be important for academic professionals to support the precepts of both leadership and management in their respective organizations. In many situations faculty could utilize administrators and professionals from other fields to perform managerial responsibilities, while they provide the leadership vision and support.

Management

Fisher, R., & Ury, W. (1983). *Getting to yes: Negotiating agreement without giving in.*

This book began as a question: What is the best way for people to deal with differences? Drawing on their backgrounds in international law and anthropology, the authors developed a practical method for negotiating agreement amicably without giving in.

The method of "principled negotiation" developed at the Harvard Negotiation Project is an excellent model for academic professionals. It suggests that you look for mutual gains and insist that results be based upon fair standards independent of the view of either side. The initial chapter of the book describes problems that require using strategies of positional bargaining. This is followed by chapters on the principles of the method: (1) separate people from the problems; (2) focus on interests, not positions; (3) invent options for mutual gain; and (4) insist on using objective criteria. The remaining sections answer questions most commonly asked about the method: What if the other side is more powerful? What if they will not play along? What if they use dirty tricks?

Since conflict is built into the multidimensional nature of academic medicine, this book should be required reading for academic physicians as they negotiate their roles and assist colleagues who are having difficulty meeting organizational or professional responsibilities. Principled negotiation can be used for both individual and group conflict management.

Jay, A. (1976). *How to run a meeting.*

In every organization, people come together in small groups at regular intervals to conduct their work. Despite the advance of electronic media and video displays, it is unlikely that face-to-face meetings will ever be replaced. This article presents the six main functions of meetings and points out why meetings become ineffective.

The author also suggests a set of guidelines to improve the effectiveness of meetings. These include: (1) a preparation phase of defining the objective, arranging the agenda, and informing members; (2) the chairman's role of directing discussion, intervening judiciously, monitoring objectives, and summarizing; (3) conducting the meeting by establishing cause of action, identifying items for information discussion and decision, time-limiting discussion, and dealing with individual behaviors and solicitation on input; and (4) follow-up with a written record and documentation of future responsibilities.

Academic physicians will probably spend over 50% of their administrative time in meetings. This article provides many valuable suggestions for making these meetings productive and time-efficient. A systematic approach for planning and conducting meetings is also a useful skill for education and research functions.

Lewis, D., & Dahl, J. O. R. (1976). *Time management in higher education administration: A case study.*

In 1974 the administrative staff in a major American university elected to participate in a self-study of their time management at their college. The eight chairpersons and directors and four deans identified 10 objectives that would help them learn more about the nature of their work.

The research methods of this self-study included the use of a carefully defined and designed code list to match the objectives and a device called the Extensor Unit that was used for self-recording each participant's behavior. The findings of the study showed that the participants did not have an accurate picture of how their time was being spent. In actuality, 68.6% of their time was spent in meetings. Time devoted to research (8.5%) was lower than estimated (21.2%). The study revealed that the participants acted on someone else's initiative over half of the time, in a planned manner, and were oriented to tasks that they felt could not be delegated. They spent approximately half of their time as administrators and devoted the rest of their time to professional responsibilities.

In the final phase of the study, the participants reviewed their personal report and developed a list of priority tasks (and the time required for them), and established a personal "time budget" for implementation.

Academic physicians are vulnerable to time mismanagement due to their multiple roles and propensity to take on more than they can reasonably accomplish in normal work hours. This study provides a detailed analysis of time allocation in an academic setting and the particular activities that cause the most stress (such as meetings, interruptions, and lack of personal time). The time organization and budgeting suggestions could be easily applied in academic medicine if faculty would analyze their roles carefully and institute some time management strategies on at least a department-wide basis.

McLaughlin, C. P. (1979). *Strategic planning and the control process at academic medical centers.*

Health care managers facing financial cutbacks must learn new skills for strategic planning, including: (1) diagnosing causes of weak claims on resources, (2) responding to the causes of those weak claims, (3) developing new coalitions at the state and local levels, and (4) maintaining credibility with the local public and professional client constituencies.

The causes of resource problems are either environmental, internal, technological, conceptual, or some combination of all of these. The author gives examples of each of these causes and points out the managers must first decide how to survive the cutbacks, then develop a strategic plan "to modify the impact of the situation on the future allocation process."

Possible responses to the causes of weak claims on resources are explored next. These include short-run changes such as stalling or bridging the onslaught of cutbacks, as well as long-range plans for changing the organization itself. The author presents examples of possible responses to each of the situations presented earlier, including environmental economic weaknesses, environmental political weaknesses, internal political inadequacies, internal managerial weaknesses, technological change, and conceptual change. The author concludes that "any given situation may involve several relative weaknesses, and the task of the manager is to develop a scenario that is appropriate to the situation."

Most academic medical centers are in the midst of budget cutbacks in several areas. Faculty must therefore become skilled in strategic planning at departmental and institutional levels.

McLaughlin, C. P., Sheldon, A., Hansen, R. C., & McIver, B. A. (1976). *Management uses of the Delphi.*

While the authors advocate face-to-face, open communication as the best way to achieve participatory decision making, policy setting, and planning in health care organizations, this requires a long-term, team-building process. They recommend using successive questionnaires (the Delphi) as an alternative approach for problem solving and planning.

The Delphi is a questionnaire that is repeated and completed anonymously. Between each administration, the results are compiled and given back to the participants so they can change their answers in light of the new formation. It is particularly useful in groups where status differences and power struggles interfere with problem solving, because opinions and suggestions are not traceable back to their owners.

The authors describe five uses of the Delphi technique in health organizations. The most common use is for predicting future events.

Another common use is to survey views and attitudes about health management. It can be used to identify problems as well as strengths and weaknesses of an organization. The Delphi is a particularly helpful mechanism for airing controversial views. The article includes a sample of several rounds of the Delphi used to identify problems in a large urban mental health center.

The Delphi method for planning and problem solving is a systematic decision-making model that academic physicians can apply in a variety of administrative situations. The process allows for a wide cross-section of input, which is a high priority among professionals. Utilizing the Delphi method will also keep academic physicians from being "reactive" decision makers. This procedure requires a certain amount of time so that information can be solicited and analyzed. This additional time to gather input and resubmit it for review could result in a more effective solution, and one that has a broad base of support.

Stone, H. (1980). *Self-management: A model for professional accountability in education.*

The influx of professionals in academic medicine has brought with it the twofold challenge of (1) allowing individuals self-expression and initiative and (2) maintaining an accountability system that keeps the organization's goals in perspective. The author has designed a method to systematically analyze and appraise academic performance, recognizing the professional values of autonomy and self-regulation. Seven basic fundamentals of self-management are: (1) visibility of departmental and individual goals; (2) objective-setting as a shared responsibility by professional and organization; (3) visibility for specific roles and activities; (4) specific evaluation based upon predetermined objectives; (5) variability in evaluation that is collected from several sources over time; (6) accountability, which reports results and (7) accepts responsibility for deficiencies and makes appropriate changes.

Stone also states that supervision in a self-management system should help people fulfill their responsibilities. Planning, analysis, appraisal, and recognition of achievements are essential supervisory functions. Peer review is also an important process in evaluating professional competence.

The application of a self-management and accountability system for academic physicians could help individual faculty to establish a performance plan for the roles of educator, researcher, clinician, and administrator. It would help them document results and establish a meaningful record of professional accomplishments. The implementation of this system requires mutual effort between faculty member and department chair. In addition, other department faculty will be involved in the peer review and/or supervision of one or more roles.

References

Aluise, J. (1982). *The organizational structure and leadership of academic family medicine departments.* University Microfilms, #8222822.

Aluise, J., & Bogdewic, S. (1984). Department management in academic family medicine. Problems and strategies from a case study investigation. *Family Practice Research, 5*(4), 207–216.

Aluise, J., Bogdewic, S., & McLaughlin, C. (1985, Winter). Organizational development in academic medicine: An educational approach.*Health Care Management Review, 10*(1), 37–43.

Aluise, J., Bogdewic, S., & Sakata, R. (1984). Organizational diagnosis for academic family medicine. *Family Medicine, 15*(6), 216–219.

Aluise, J., Kirkman-Liff, B., & Neely, G. (1981). Administration in family medicine education—an academic quandary. *Family Practice, 12*(2), 249–257.

American Medical Association. (published biannualy). *The environment of medicine; Report of the Council of Long Range Planning and Development.* Chicago: Author.

Argyris, C. (1957). *Personality and organization.* New York: Harper & Row.

Berman, P., & McLaughlin, M. (1973). *Implementing innovations: Revisions for an agenda for a study of change agent programs in education.* Itasca, IL: Peacock Publishers.

Cope, R. G. (1978). *Strategic policy planning.* (Littleton, CO: Ireland Educational Group.

Delbecq, A. L., & Gill, S. L. (1985, Winter). Justice as a prelude to teamwork in medical centers. *Health Care Management Review, 10*(1), 45–51.

Drucker, P. (1974a). *Business purpose and business mission in management tasks and responsibilities.* New York: Harper & Row.

Drucker, P. F. (1974b). New templates for today's organizations. *Harvard Business Review, 52,* 45–53.

Ebert, R. H., & Brown, S. S. (1983). Academic health centers. *New England Journal of Medicine, 308*(2), 1200–1207.

Fisher, R., & Ury, W. (1983). *Getting to yes: Negotiating agreement without giving in.* New York: Penguin Books.

Giaguita, J. (1973). The process of organizational change in schools. In F. W. Kerlinger (Ed.), *Review of research in education.* Itasca, IL: Peacock Publishers.

Greiner, L. E. (1972, July–August). Evolution and revolution as organizations grow. *Harvard Business Review, 50,* 37–46.

Gross, N., Gianuinta, J., & Berstein, M. (1971). *Implementing organizational innovations: A sociological analysis of planned educational change.* New York: Basic Books.

Havelock, R., & Havelock, M. (1973). *Training for change agents: A guide to the design of training programs in education and other fields.* Ann Arbor: Institute for Social Research, University of Michigan.

Jay, A. (1976, March–April). How to run a meeting. *Harvard Business Review, 54,* 43–57.

Katz, D., & Kahn, R. (1966). *The social psychology of organizations.* New York: John Wiley & Sons.

Korok, M. (1983). Medical education: Prospectus interrupta. *Journal of the American Medical Association, 249,* 1–2.

Lewis, D., & Dahl, J. O. R. (1976). Time management in higher education administration: A case study. *Higher Education, 5,* 49–66.

Likert, R. (1961). *New patterns of management.* New York: McGraw-Hill.

Lorange, P., & Vancil, R. F. (1976, September–October). How to design a strategic planning system. *Harvard Business Review, 54,* 75.

McCall, M. W., Jr. (1982). *Leadership and the professional* (technical report). Greensboro, NC: Center for Creative Leadership.

McGaghie, W., & Frey, J. J. (Eds.). (1986). *Handbook for academic physicians.* New York: Springer-Verlag.

McLaughlin, C. P. (1979). *Strategic planning and the control process at academic medical centers.* Washington, DC: Association of American Medical Colleges.

McLaughlin, C. P., Sheldon, A., Hansen, R. C., & McIver, B. A. (1976, Spring). Management uses of the Delphi. *Health Care Management Review, 1,* 51–62.

Miller, D. (1986). *Managing professionals in research and development.* San Francisco: Jossey-Bass.

Mintzberg, H. (1979). *The structuring of organizations.* Englewood Cliffs, NJ: Prentice-Hall

Nash, D. (1987). *Future practice alternatives in medicine.* New York: Igaku-Shoin Medical Publishers.

Peters, T., & Waterman, R. (1982). *In search of excellence.* New York: Harper & Row.

Pfeiffer, J., & Jones, J. (Eds.). (published yearly). *Handbook for group facilitators.* La Jolla, CA: University Associates.

Prince, G. (1982, July–August). Creative meetings through power sharing. *Harvard Business Review, 60,* 47–54.

Project planning exercise. Plymouth, MI: Human Synergistics.

Rogers, D. E., & Blendon, R. J. (1978). The academic medical center: A stressed American institution. *New England Journal of Medicine, 298*(17), 940–950.

Rothlisberger, F., & Dickson, W. (1939). *Management and the worker.* Cambridge, MA: Harvard University Press.

Schein, E. (1978). *Career dynamics: Matching individual and organizational needs.* Reading, MA: Addison-Wesley.

Schmidt, W., & Tannenbaum, R. (1960, November–December). Management of differences. *Harvard Business Review*, 107–115.

Self, T. (1980, March). *The institutionalization of family medicine education.* Publication Number HRA 81–18. Silver Spring, MD: U.S. Department of Health and Human Resources.

Sorkin, A. (1986). *Health care and the changing economic environment.* Lexington, MA: Lexington Books.

Stone, H. (1980). *Self-management: A model for professional accountability in education.* Unpublished report, Educational Resources Center for Health Services, University of Wisconsin.

Strasser, S. (1983, Winter). The effective application of contingency theory in health settings: Problems and recommended solutions. *Health Care Management Review, 8,* 15–23.

Thomas, L. (1983). *The youngest science.* New York: Viking Press.

Weisbord, M. (1976, Spring). Why organizational development hasn't worked in medical centers. *Health Care Management Review, 1,* 45–52.

Weisbord, M. R. (1978). *Organization diagnosis: A workbook of theory and practice.* Reading, MA: Addison-Wesley.

Weisbord, M., Lawrence, P., & Charns, M. (1978). Three dilemmas of the academic medical centers. *Journal of Applied Behavioral Science, 14*(3), 284–304.

Wilson, M. P., & McLaughlin, C. (1984). *Leadership and management in academic medicine.* San Francisco: Jossey-Bass.

Zaleznik, A. (1977, May–June). Managers and leaders: Are they different? *Harvard Business Review, 55,* 67–78.

CHAPTER 5

Research Domain

Introduction to the Domain

Only a century ago, research was limited to part-time activities of a select small number of individuals working in very limited settings. Today, thousands of individuals pursue research careers that are financed by government and the private sector. Universities represent a segment of our society that has a primary mission to support researchers and research activity. The successful academician must evaluate the role that research will take in his or her academic career.

The word *research* has its origins in a term that means "to search thoroughly." *Experiment* refers to an operation carried out under controlled conditions in order to discover an unknown. These definitions emphasize two key elements in this domain: first, that research actively pursues the uncovering of new facts; and second, that people who engage in research do so in a systematic way in controlled situations.

Medical science has evolved in a complex fashion that prevents a single research model from covering all relevant research questions. The research traditions within medicine are varied and can include basic science, clinical science, epidemiology, the behavioral and social sciences, and health services research, to name just a few. In recent years many specialities in medicine have begun to assess their own research accomplishments and to set research agendas for the coming years. Perkoff (1981) classified five main types of research ranging from the content and delivery of medical care to cross-cultural studies. He warned that although the experimental model may fit many of our problems and probably represents the gold standard of research, different methodologies will be necessary to address questions that are important to ask. Thus, it seems we should not expect a single research paradigm to adequately serve the diversity of research questions in a discipline as eclectic as primary care medicine.

Definition of the Research Domain

Our task with this curriculum, therefore, is to define the research domain in a way that accommodates both the diverse and common skills that faculty need in order to generate and use research knowledge in an academic community. We have done this by examining the general premises and process steps of the scientific method (Butterfield, 1960). This method is the foundation for all the research traditions listed above.

This method sets forth a set of rules for studying phenomena of interest and has as its goals objectivity, empirical verification, contribution to knowledge, and publication or presentation of results. The scientific method is, in a sense, the honor code that binds the research community and serves as the standard for development of knowledge.

The general steps of the scientific method are described by True (1983) as:

1. *Specify Goals.* The purpose of a research project should be clear. A research goal is chosen and kept firmly in mind throughout the study so that all subsequent efforts focus on it. At the end of the project, the goal is reviewed and the results evaluated with reference to it. A research goal is often revised in light of what has been done by others.
2. *Review the Literature.* All good research builds on previous investigations. A thorough familiarity with the work already done is mandatory in order to learn what has been accomplished, to profit by other people's mistakes and triumphs, and to see what needs exist. The researcher reads not only the reports of research projects but also the relevant theory. The literature review affects the research goals and the methods chosen.
3. *Design the Study.* The study design is the concrete plan that guides decisions regarding how data will be gathered, what types of instruments and measures will be employed, and how data will be analyzed and interpreted. A well-conceived and coherent study design enables other researchers to replicate investigations in new settings or with new subject populations.

4. *Invite Scrutiny.* Peer scrutiny (in addition to the literature review) affects both the research goals and the methods of measuring and recording data. At every stage of a research project the opinions and advice of colleagues should be solicited. Publication of research is the ultimate invitation to scrutiny. Regardless of specialized interest, all fellow scientists can help a researcher by critiquing the work, suggesting improvements, and asking questions.

This domain, therefore, is based on literature supporting the scientific method, as drawn from the areas of epidemiology, biostatistics, experimental psychology, and the qualitative inquiry methods currently seen in educational psychology. Kuhn (1964) sets the stage by describing the evolution of scientific paradigms. Methods of reviewing and interpreting the literature are presented by Cooper (1984), Gehlbach (1988), Riegelman (1981), Sackett, Hanes, and Tugwell (1985), and Light and Pillemer (1984). Methodological skills for quantitative research are well taught in texts by O'Brien and Shampo (1981), Colton (1982), Feinstein (1977), Schefler (1984), and others (Godfrey, 1985a, b; Levy & Lemeshow, 1980; Marks, 1982a, b; Niemi & Sullivan, 1980–1985; Young, Bresnit, & Strom, 1983). Epidemiological techniques are specifically supplied by Kelsey, Thompson, and Evans (1986) and Kleinbaum, Kupper, and Morgenstern (1982). Procedures for qualitative research are supplied by Patton (1975) and Guba (1978). In addition, the skills of managing research are detailed in McGaghie and Frey (1986) and Berg, Gordon, and Cherkin (1986).

Rationale for Including Research in the Curriculum

Who should, or can, conduct research? Only the full-time faculty member in a research-oriented university? The faculty member in a community hospital? The preceptor or practitioner in the "practice lab?" As readers probably realize, members in our discipline disagree, sometimes heatedly, about this issue. Perhaps more than for any other domain, the rationale for research skills engages us immediately in questions of relevance for particular faculty members. Research in the abstract is undoubtedly essential for any discipline to grow. But which faculty are most responsible for the discipline? Why? Can traditional models of research effort (i.e., the single investigator with federal or foundation dollars) continue to guide research development today?

Although readers will have to resolve these questions individually for their own setting, we believe that all practitioners, all teachers,

and certainly all researchers need a foundation in some research competencies. For example, without some background in research, it would
be impossible to engage in continuing self-education; one would not
be able to critically screen and analyze the onslaught of research articles. In many cases the conclusions seen in a series of topic-related
articles are contradictory. Only the reader with basic skills in evaluating a research article can make informed decisions about the merit
of any research finding and whether it justifies changing clinical
practices.

Clinical faculty similarly need to continually update themselves
on medical and education topics. They are responsible for articulat-
ing the literature from many areas to students. They serve as primary
role models; they must believe in and practice the integration of practice and research. Their familiarity with the literature should extend
to conceptual grasp of the research process. Because the discipline
of medicine is so large, the problem of remaining current calls for some
very sophisticated reading strategies.

Finally, for the stability and growth of our discipline, we believe
that all of us must accept some level of responsibility for investigating and furthering our understanding of the premises, truths, and
theories that guide medical science. Clearly, the lion's share of the
responsibility will fall to full-time faculty members in research universities. This is not to say that others will not make numerous and significant contributions. They will. It is appropriate, however, to expect
the faculty who are in institutions whose major mission is research,
and who are surrounded by research colleagues and resources, to bear
most of this responsibility. Primary care faculty must promote, from
within their ranks, a force that is committed to theorizing, hypothesiz-
ing, and leading research efforts that are vital to our field.

How the Domain Has Been Structured

The research domain can be divided into three components that reflect
the general scientific method and explain the interrelation of basic
competencies (see Table 5.1). These components indicate that the successful researcher understands the content of the research topic; knows
how to select and apply appropriate methods in answering research
questions; and is effective in managing resources required for research
initiatives.

The first component, content knowledge, concerns the individual
research interests of faculty and the necessary mastery of information related to it, such as significant lines of research, primary concepts and constructs, traditional tools or approaches used, and current

findings. Because research interests are different for each faculty member, no attempt to discuss content prerequisites has been made. Rather, it is presumed that faculty will pursue this with their colleagues and mentors and on their own. (The skills for doing so have been enumerated in this chapter.)

The component in the center, methodological skills, encompasses a full range of relevant methods. Faculty researchers are not expected to learn all of the skills related to all the research paradigms that potentially apply to their specialty, but they *do* need grounding in the basic scientific method and related quantitative research skills, for these competencies undergird all research paradigms. Researchers will then need to acquire advanced skills in the unique methods and approaches that fit their own research questions.

The central component deals with the problematic issue of basic versus advanced research skills by specifying a range of competencies in the following pages. These skills have been listed in ascending order (from basic to advanced) under each subarea of the domain. Readers will see that the basic competencies are written in more detail than the advanced because these, we feel, should be required of everyone, and it is not possible to write competencies for every conceivable methodology at the advanced level. Instead, advanced competencies are stated generically, and faculty are expected to relate them to their own research areas.

The third component in Table 5.1 represents the practical skills of conducting research, such as managing personnel, meeting deadlines, and budgeting.

Assumptions Made in Constructing the Domain

In introducing this domain we presented the scientific method as a philosophic foundation to research. In addition to this bias, if you will, we confess to holding five additional premises. First, a strong foundation in one's content area is prerequisite to investigating it through the research process. Too often we jump into a study without really knowing the literature on our topic. Providing support to this first premise, the Survey of Department Chairs and Residency Directors (Schmitz, Bland & Stritter, 1986; see Appendix) identified "accessing and reading literature relevant to one's special interests" as the most essential skill in the research domain.

A second premise is that all researchers must master certain basic methodological skills. Research that does not have a clear plan for conducting the study or precise definition of terms, for example, is headed for certain doom. This lack of methodologic know-how seems to be a common problem for inexperienced faculty investigators.

The third premise is that successful research requires more than just a well-conceived question and research plan. The management of a research project requires skills few people consider during the formal training. The administration of a budget, research personnel, and facilities are only a few of the issues an investigator must address. Many good research studies fail because of faulty management.

The fourth premise is that while many of the competencies can be acquired through self-instruction or course work, there is no good substitute for participating in research projects with experienced investigators. The process of active involvement with consultants and mentors is possibly the best method for solidifying research expertise. Reading and observing will provide knowledge, but only through active participation does one learn the finer skills of research. Because of the mission of research universities, most successful mentoring occurs there. Most new faculty who seek careers as researchers will find it necessary to spend 2 to 5 years at a research university in order to develop their skills to a competitive level.

The final premise is a caution. Many disciplines have a significant number of formally trained researchers who are not conducting research. Bland and Schmitz (1986) found that skills and knowledge alone will not make a successful researcher. Researchers need support not only in terms of protected time, but in terms of supportive organizational values and attitudes. Attitudes and values are acquired from sustained interactions with significant others, such as mentors, advisors, and departmental research leaders. These organizational factors and socialization experiences (discussed in the Professional Academic Skills Domain, Chapter 2) seem to be as important as any set of competencies in determining who will be a successful researcher. Individuals who are committed to developing research skills for their faculty must have a specific plan for protecting enough of their time and for providing adequate research mentors and teachers or the program will meet with known fatal barriers to successful research. This caution cannot be stated too strongly.

Goals and Competencies

Listed below are the goals and competencies for the research domain. This list represents a spectrum of knowledge and skills required of faculty in research; it is not broken down by institution or faculty type.

For suggestions on how to identify relevant subsets of competencies for preceptors, non-tenure-track, and tenure-track faculty see Chapter 7.

These goals and competencies were prepared by the content expert after engaging in an extensive literature review, meeting with physician liaisons and advisory committee members, reviewing the results of three surveys, and discussing the domain with the other authors. The competencies are presented according to each subarea of the domain as illustrated in Table 5.1

Content Knowledge: Reading the Research Literature

GOAL 11.0: To access and critically read the research literature in medicine, education, and other domains.

GOAL 12.0: To understand theory and empirical findings in one's own research area.

The information explosion in medicine presents faculty with an enormous challenge. Screening, reading, and evaluating the medical literature are absolutely essential skills for all faculty, whether they practice full-time or have research appointments. For the clinician preparing to engage in formal investigations, reading and assessing research articles are critical preliminary steps. Researchers need to have a clear understanding of the problem and how it has been traditionally studied before they begin the research process. Knowledge

TABLE 5.1 Subareas in the Research Domain

Content Knowledge
- Reading the clinical and theoretical research literature critically
- Understanding theory and findings in areas of interest

Methodological Skills
- Defining purpose, hypothesis, and variables
- Selecting research design
- Data collection and analysis
- Interpreting results
- Publication*

Management Skills
- Managing time, personnel, budgets

---

* Publication of research results is presented in the Written Communication domain (Chapter 6).

of the literature is crucial because it guides the remainder of the researcher process. For this reason, command of one's content area stands as the most important prerequisite to acquiring methodological skills.

Faculty should be able to:

11.1. Use appropriate resources (libraries, computers) to complete literature searches; be familiar with available software packages to search literature (MEDLINE, Grateful Med)

11.2. Evaluate a research article critically

12.1. Identify an area of interest in a given body of literature

12.2. Identify experts in that area of interest

12.3. Explain (in a general way) the importance of theory to research

12.4. Relate specific questions of interest to underlying theory

12.5. Pursue an area of interest over an extended period of time, remaining current in pertinent literature

12.6. Recognize the classic studies, traditional designs, common forms of measurement, common variables, and common methodological problems related to one's own research content

12.7. Critically synthesize the literature relevant to one's own research question

12.8. Identify conferences and professional organizations that focus on one's own research area

Methodological Skills: Research Purpose, Hypotheses, Variables, and Operational Definitions

GOAL 13.0: To formulate a research question and operationalize variables.

Essential to any research study is a direct statement of the problem and purpose. When the purpose is ambiguous it is impossible to develop a clear research plan and results cannot be interpreted. Successful researchers learn to state the problem and questions to be investigated in such a way that their audiences can understand what the study will accomplish. Too often this preplanning is ignored and confusion over definitions of important terms leads to weak or unsuccessful research.

Faculty should be able to:

13.1. Identify a problem or general question to investigate

13.2. Refine the problem so it can be investigated

13.3. Establish a clear purpose to the research

13.4. Translate the general question into specific hypotheses, recognizing the difference between research, null, and alternative hypotheses

13.5. Define variables and terms operationally

13.6. Recognize the difference between independent and dependent variables when applicable

13.7. Determine how each variable will be measured, recognizing different levels of measurement (nominal, ordinal, interval, ratio)

13.8. Evaluate the reliability and validity of a given measurement

13.9. Evaluate variables and their measurement in one's area of research and know how they compare to other similar measures

Methodological Skills: Research Design and Procedures

GOAL 14.0: To design descriptive and/or explanatory studies.

The research design is the blueprint for how the research question will be studied. It describes how subjects are entered into the study and how and when the data are collected. Specific research design decisions are reflected by the kind of research question the investigator selects.

Unfortunately for the novice researcher, selecting a research design to match the research question is not a simple task. Furthermore, even within focused research topics there are numerous design choices to be made, depending on how the researcher wants to address the problem. Different designs can be applied to the same research question, but each has the potential to shed a different light on the problem and leads to different sorts of conclusions.

Researchers must become familiar with a variety of different research designs and understand the advantages and disadvantages of each for their own research questions. For example, a case-control study requires a very different design from a true experimental study, despite the fact that they are both considered explanatory research. Ethnography and case studies are both examples of descriptive research, but each has its own unique set of rules and regulations that determine how each is to be conducted. Regardless of the research paradigm one accepts, careful attention to the design of that study is essential for drawing meaningful conclusions.

Faculty should be able to:

14.1. Categorize research designs (e.g., observational vs. interventional, and prospective vs. retrospective)

14.2. State the purpose, strengths, and limitations of each design

14.3. Compare major types of studies, such as case reports, case controls, cross-sectional, longitudinal, and epidemiological studies, clinical trials, survey studies, field research, and evaluation studies

14.4. Explain important threats to internal and external validity applicable in each design

14.5. State the relationship between the chosen research design, the type of data collected, and the necessary statistical techniques

14.6. Prepare for and use consultation from design specialists

14.7. Thoroughly analyze the dominant research designs used in one's special area of study

14.8. Recognize sources of error in one's study and methods to minimize error when possible

Methodological Skills: Data Collection and Analysis

GOAL 15.0: To collect and analyze data.

Good planning in research always anticipates how the data will be analyzed. For cross-sectional and longitudinal studies, statistical analysis is the mechanism for determining if research hypotheses are confirmed or not. Secondary analysis techniques help summarize large amounts of quantitative data so that study results can be communicated in a meaningful fashion. Just as an investigator must select the appropriate resource design to match the research question, so must he or she select appropriate analytic techniques to match the research design used and type of data collected.

Accurate data analysis is a necessary step if valid conclusions are to be drawn. Data analysis and research design considerations require many investigators to seek assistance from consultants because these components of research are highly technical and beyond the scope of training for many physicians. Also, computers have become an essential and important tool for researchers. All new investigators should understand in what ways a computer can assist them in managing and conducting a research project.

Faculty should be able to:

15.1. Distinguish inferential from descriptive statistics

15.2. Determine the universe, population, appropriate sample, sample size, and appropriate sampling technique for a given study

15.3. Understand basic statistical concepts such as: statistical significance, mean, median, mode, standard deviations, standard error, prevalence rate, incidence rate, and p-value

15.4. Understand commonly used statistical tests, such as chi-square, t-test, analysis of variance, correlations, and multiple regression

15.5. Construct a plan for managing data files and for analyzing those data according to their level of measurement and the research design

15.6. Be familiar with available statistical packages (e.g., SPSS, SAS, BMD) to direct computer personnel in what analysis to use and what related decisions must be made (e.g., how to handle missing data)

15.7. Interpret printouts on common analyses from available statistical packages (listed above) for one's research area

15.8. Understand how to graphically summarize and communicate data in an efficient manner (e.g., histogram, bar graph, pie chart, frequency curve)

15.9. Report results correctly and be able to cite strengths and limitations of the study based on the data

15.10. Prepare for and use consultation from computer analysts and statisticians

15.11. Understand more advanced statistical tests used in one's research area, such as discriminant analysis, principal components analysis, and multiple logistic analysis

Methodological Skills: Data Evaluation and Discussion

GOAL 16.0: To evaluate and discuss study findings.

Data evaluation requires interpreting and judging the research results in light of the original questions and related research literature. Given the specific motivation for conducting the study, the investigator evaluates what new knowledge has been acquired.

Faculty should be able to:

16.1. Explain the outcome of given analyses in terms of the originally stated hypothesis

16.2. Conduct additional literature review as needed to elaborate upon findings and their implications for a given body of research

16.3. Integrate the research findings into the existing literature by discussing what is known, unknown, and requires further study

16.4. Express appropriate cautions in interpreting results, and base these cautions on methodological and theoretical conditions

16.5. Place one's study in the context of existing research and justify how it contributes to important questions in the area

Management Skills: Conducting a Research Project

GOAL 17.0: To conduct and manage research projects.

Even the best-planned research study can fail if it does not attend to administrative details. Investigators must ensure that deadlines are met, that personnel are given clearly stated tasks and protocols, and that budgets are kept. Only occasionally does formal research training offer training in project management. Too often, poor management results in stalled or abandoned projects. Because textbooks and courses overlook these competencies, many novice researchers do not acquire administrative skills in research until a project has suffered from poor management.

Faculty should be able to:

17.1. Develop plans for implementing a study, including timeline, budget, requirements for personnel, facilities, and supplies.

17.2. Identify appropriate funding sources (local, state, national)

17.3. Identify faculty collaborators from within and outside the discipline who can offer guidance to the project

17.4. Hire, manage, and evaluate personnel involved with a study

17.5. Prepare and submit required reports, budget requests, and other administrative documents

17.6. Secure permission from human subjects, research, and other institutional review committees and boards

17.7. Implement and direct a research project

17.8. Prepare a research proposal suitable for submission in one's research area

Courses, Strategies, and Resources

Listed below are suggested courses, strategies, and resources for teaching the competencies and achieving the goals of the Research domain (Competencies to be achieved by each course or other activity are listed by number after each description.) These activities and sources cover the full range of skills identified in Table 2.1 under "Research;" they are not keyed to specific faculty types of particular institutions. For guidelines on how to select and combine courses in this (and other) domain(s) for preceptors, non-tenure-track, and tenure-track faculty, see Implementation Models, Chapter 8.

301. INTRODUCTION TO MEDICAL RESEARCH (Nine 3-hour sessions)

This introductory seminar describes the discipline of research and reviews the different research traditions and paradigms found in medical research. Its purpose is to orient new researchers to the history and organization of medical research and to help them understand the many ways these topics can be studied. Also included in the seminar is a component on the philosophy of science. Here participants are oriented to the historical and philosophical perspectives in research and the logic behind theory- and paradigm-building.

During the seminar, experienced researchers lead discussions on different research issues. For example, a clinical epidemiologist is invited to discuss how an epidemiologist engages in research. He or she outlines the research questions, methodologies, classic studies, and journals that epidemiologists read. The same format is followed by researchers representing clinical trials, medical ethnography, behavioral research, survey research, health services research, and other topics of interest to new researchers. In addition, participants receive material summarizing each orientation.

Competencies: 12.1, 12.3–12.6.

Suggested Resource Material

Suitable resource material for this and other literature/content knowledge-related courses can be found following course #304.

302. ASSESSING THE RESEARCH LITERATURE (Four 3-hour sessions)

This course teaches participants how to critically analyze the research literature found in primary care research journals. The course focuses on the essential components of a research article and ways to evaluate the merits and weaknesses of those components. Understanding the purpose, structure, and methods of a research article is a prerequisite to designing original research.

Strategies

1. Presenter provides participants with a worksheet designed to assess each type of research article (e.g., clinical trial, retrospective study, cross-sectional)
2. Participants read an original article and apply the worksheet to the article
3. Participants lead a discussion critiquing the strengths and weaknesses of the study and offer suggestions for improving the investigation.

Suggested Topics

- Anatomy of an article
- Study design
- Instrumentation and measurement
- Analysis of results
- Risk assessment
- Cause and effect relationships
- Drawing conclusions

Competencies: 12.2–12.6 and 11.1–11.2.

303. HOW TO USE A LIBRARY (Two half-day workshops)

Participants learn how to use the resources of their hospital or university library and to stay current in their special areas of interest. They are introduced to the advantages of using the computer to facilitate the research process from literature searches to project management and analysis.

Strategies

1. Provide an overview of what the library can offer

2. Demonstrate for participants how they can obtain answers to their specific content questions from staff librarians
3. Participants conduct computerized medical literature searches in their content area using an existing data base such as MEDLINE, Catline, ERIC

Suggested Topics

- Understanding the logic of Index Medicus
- How to order a MEDLINE search
- How to order a methodological search
- How to use a bibliography of medical reviews
- How to use the Science Citation Index

Competencies: 11.1–11.2, 12.3–12.7.

304. CONDUCTING AN INTEGRATED RESEARCH REVIEW (Two half-day workshops)

Participants who have already completed courses 301, 302, and 303 are now prepared to do the following: examine multiple articles in one topic area; evaluate the contribution of each for understanding that topic; and, finally, integrate those evaluations into a more comprehensive statement on the progress of that research area. Conducting a literature review and drawing meaningful conclusions from existing articles is a skill that is practiced thoroughly in this workshop.

Strategies

1. Presenters provide essential steps in conducting a research review
2. Participants apply the review steps to their content area in a homework assignment
3. Participants receive a model for structuring the components of their research review
4. At the end of the session, participants submit their own organizational structure for articles and major conclusions drawn from the collection of articles
5. Participants formulate two to three researchable questions appropriate to the above review

Suggested Topics

- The stages of research reviews

- Formulating the problem for review
- Research review coding sheet
- Hand and computerized literature searches
- Issues in research synthesis
- A format for reporting the integrative research review

Competencies: 11.1, 12.1, 12.5, 12.7.

Suggested Resource Material

For complete citations, see the Reference Section at the end of this chapter. Also check the Annotated Bibliography for fuller descriptions.

Alguire, P., Henry, R., Massa, M., & Lienhart, K. (1986). *Power reading: Critical appraisal of the medical literature.* A packaged course for teaching appraisal of research literature.
Butterfield, H. (1960). *The origins of modern science.*
Cooper, H. M. (1984). *The integrative research review: A systematic approach.*
Gehlbach, S. H. (1988). *Interpreting the medical literature: A clinician's guide* (2nd ed.).
Geyman, J. P., & Berg, A. O. (1984). 1974–1983: Analysis of an evolving literature base.
Goldman, L., Mushlin, A. I., & Lee, K. L. (1986). Using medical data bases for clinical research.
Hayden, G. F., Kramer, M. S., & Horowitz, R. I. (1982). The case-control study.
Huth, E. J. (1986). The primary care research environment.
National Library of Medicine. (1985). *The basics of searching MEDLINE: A guide for the health professional.*
Norman, G. R., & Streiner, D. L. (1986). *PDQ statistics.*
Riegelman, R. K. (1981). *Studying a study and testing a test: How to read the medical literature.*
Sacket, D. L., Hanes, R. B., & Tugwell, P. (1985). *Clinical epidemiology: A basic science for clinical medicine.*

305. RESEARCH PLANNING SEMINAR (Three half-day workshops)

A seminar that takes participants step-by-step through the research planning process. The end product is a very specific research plan that serves as a guide for implementing a research study.

Strategies

1. Presenters describe common strategies for identifying research questions

2. Participants develop a research question of interest to them
3. Research experts provide presentations on the fundamentals of research planning
4. Participants complete a research workbook in which they detail how they will complete each step of the research process
5. Participants are assigned a research advisor who is knowledgeable in the content and methods selected for the research topic. This advisor provides assistance throughout the first research project.
6. Homework assignments are completed each week and discussed the following week during class
7. Participants formally present their designs and plans for implementation to the faculty and other participants

Suggested Topics

- Focusing a research question
- Developing operational definitions
- Selecting a research design
- Identifying instruments and outcome measures
- Developing a flow chart for data collection
- Designing implementation procedures
- Budgeting the research project

Competencies: 13.1–13.8, 14.1–14.8.

Suggested Resource Material

Suitable resource material for this and other methods-related activities can be found following course #311.

306. INTRODUCTION TO DATA MANAGEMENT (Two half-day workshops)

Participants learn to develop procedures and forms for data collection, organization, and preparation for later analysis and reporting. Participants should recognize that nearly all data management is facilitated with a computer and that they need to become familiar with computer facilities and personnel at their institution.

Strategies

1. Presenters provide strategies and frameworks for organizing data collection

2. Participants develop a specific plan for organizing study data into a usable form
3. Participants interact with personnel who understand the relationship between data management and data analysis using computers and software packages

Competencies: 13.7, 14.6 and 15.2.

307. INTRODUCTION TO STATISTICAL ANALYSIS (Three half-day workshops)

This workshop offers participants a decision key for understanding fundamental questions that enter into the selection of appropriate fundamental statistical procedures.

Strategies

1. Statisticians present basic questions to ask in determining appropriate analysis techniques.
2. Participants apply the decision key to new research problems by critiquing journal article procedures and analyses
3. Participants select best analysis techniques for their own research projects

Suggested Topics

- Distinguishing inferential from descriptive statistics
- Understanding the purpose of statistical analysis
- Interpreting statistical results
- Distinguishing the most frequently used statistical tests and criteria for using each

Competencies: 15.1–15.8.

308. ADVANCED METHODS SKILL TRAINING (Variable time)

After completing the core research seminar and workshops, participants pursue advanced research methods courses appropriate to their project. At this point in the training, summer short courses may provide the most practical means for quickly acquiring specific skills. Most research universities, medical schools, and schools of public health offer special summer coursework for professionals. With the assistance of the advisor, participants identify seminars and courses that provide them with relevant training.

Competencies: 12.8, 13.9, 14.7, and 15.11.

309. INDEPENDENT RESEARCH PROJECT (Variable time)

The major outcome of the research curriculum is a completed research study. Faculty members should be expected to spend a significant amount of time implementing and managing their studies. Research advisors should meet regularly with the faculty participants to make sure the study is managed successfully and that the researcher has the necessary resources to complete the study according to plan. Although estimates of time vary significantly, most research projects require a minimum of 20% of the investigator's time for the duration of the program.

Even after successfully completing a study, researchers need additional time to acquire an in-depth understanding of their content area. They may need highly selected coursework or other planned experiences to further their development. For example, working in a geriatric assessment center or substance abuse clinic are experiences that would illuminate a research interest in those areas.

We would like to emphasize that selecting a research advisor represents a particularly important step in developing research competence. In addition to advising, this individual serves as a research and all-around role model who transmits skills, knowledge, and appropriate attitudes to the new faculty member during implementation of the study. As the novice researcher becomes more skilled, the advisor role will typically be replaced by colleagues and research associates.

Competencies: 14.6, 14.7, 15.4–15.11, 16.1–16.5, 17.1–17.8.

310. RESEARCH SEMINARS (Six half-days)

If possible, the Research Seminars should run concurrently with participants' Independent Research Projects (#309). Scheduled as periodic, informal meetings, these sessions bring participants and advisors together to discuss common research problems and questions. Each member reports on his or her progress since the previous seminar, then receives feedback and suggestions from the group. There are no prepared lectures or topic, although certain subjects may be addressed, didactically, in some detail.

Competencies: All for goals 11–17, also 24.1–24.2.

311. FORMAL COURSEWORK IN RESEARCH DESIGN AND ANALYSIS (Variable time)

The best way for novice researchers to learn statistics and research methodology is to enroll in university courses. Formal coursework and disciplined study provide the foundation in research methodology as well as access to teachers with advice on state-of-the-art techniques and a network of other researchers. While a degree program may not be necessary, formal coursework clearly expedites the development of research skills.

Competencies: 13.1–13.9, 14.1–14.8, 15.1–15.11, 16.1–16.5.

312. RESEARCH DAY (One day simulated research conference)

As a final requirement for completion of the curriculum, participants formally present the findings of their research projects to an audience of faculty and other researchers. Participants should have guidelines to follow for their presentations that simulate a research conference. These guidelines cover:

1. Submission of an abstract
2. Using audiovisual materials for display of data
3. Summarizing the study in a research paper
4. Responding to questions and comments from the audience
5. Receiving verbal and written critiques from seminar discussants

Competencies: 12.8, 16.1–16.5.

313. RESEARCH NETWORK (Variable time)

This seminar is designed to bring together academic physicians from university and community settings to collaborate on research projects. It does this by introducing them to the network concept and philosophy and by explaining how it operates. Research-oriented faculty in need of data bases and/or patient populations design studies to which practice-oriented faculty contribute primarily by collecting data. Once in the network, faculty spend varying amounts of time on studies. The network can be very valuable to the nontenured faculty member whose time for and interest in research is limited but who wishes to gain some research experience.

Competencies: 12.8, 17.2.–17.3, 24.2–24.4.

Suggested Resource Material

Ahlgren, A. (1983). *Practical data analysis with SPSS.* (Package of 12 videotapes for using and interpreting SPSS)

Cuddy, P. G., Elenbaas, R. M., & Elenbaas, J. K. (1983). Evaluating the medical literature, Part I: Abstract, introduction, methods.

Elenbaas, J. K., Cuddy, P. G., & Elenbaas, R. M. (1983). Evaluating the medical literature, Part III: Results and discussion.

Elenbaas, R. M., Elenbaas, J. K., & Cuddy, P. G. (1983). Evaluating the medical literature, Part II: Statistical analysis.

Fletcher, R. H., Fletcher, S. W., Wagner, E. H. (1988). *Clinical epidemiology: The essentials* (2nd ed.).

The Foundation Center. (1979). *The foundation directory* (7th ed.).

Geyman, J. P. (1980). Health services research: A crucial and underfunded need.

Green, L. A., et al. (1984). The ambulatory sentinel practice network: Purpose, methods, and policies.

Hall, M. (1977). *Developing skills in proposal writing* (2nd ed.).

Henry, R. C., Massa, M. D., & Ogle, K. S. (1985). *Planning a research study.*

Henry, R. C., & Zivick, J. D. (1986). Principles of survey research.

Kramer, H. C., & Thierman, S. (1987). *How many subjects? Statistical power analysis in research.*

Krathwohl, D. R. (1966). *How to prepare a research proposal.*

Marcus, A. C., & Crane, L. A. (1986). Telephone surveys in public health research.

Marks, R. G. (1982). *Analyzing research data: The basics of biomedical research methodology.*

Marks, R. G. (1982). *Designing a research project: The basics of biomedical research methodology.*

Masterman, L. E. (1978). *The applicant's guide to successful grantsmanship.*

McGraw-Hill. (1978). *McGraw-Hill's guide to health grants and contracts.*

Moses, L. E. (1985). Statistical concepts fundamental to investigations.

Perkoff, G. T. (1981). Research in family medicine: Classification, direction and costs.

U.S. Department of Health and Human Services. (1986). *NIH guide for grants and contracts.*

U.S. Government Printing Office (1985). *Update to the catalog of federal domestic assistance.*

Washington report on medicine and health. (1985).

Young, M. J., Bresnitz, E. A., & Strom, B. L. (1983). Sample size nomogram for interpreting negative clinical studies.

Rationale for the Domain Design

This domain model is built on the premise that different faculty groups will need different sets of skills in order to be successful in research. Results from the survey of residency directors and department chairs, for example (see Appendix), told us that residency directors and department chairs did not expect preceptors and non-tenure-track faculty to be knowledgeable on research principles or to engage in active research. Rather, expectations for these faculty focused on keeping current in their medical knowledge and accessing literature relevant to their special areas of practice and other faculty needs

Interestingly, these expectations seem inconsistent with the frequently held view that the research laboratory of the primary care physician is the practice setting itself (Geyman, 1978). If the practice is to be the laboratory, then physicians who conduct research in those practices must be trained in formal inquiry methods. Primarily for this reason, we feel that just being able to read research literature is not quite sufficient for preceptors and non-tenure-track faculty (see Chapter 2). Because the research efforts of nonuniversity faculty have contributed to the growth of new medical knowledge and will continue to do so, we recommend optional active research experiences for these faculty groups.

For faculty who have tenure-track appointments at predominantly research universities, we suggest formal research coursework available through the university. At most universities these courses can be found in a school of public health or college of social science or educational psychology. Most programs that offer doctoral-level training also offer a wide variety of research courses.

Faculty who pursue research as a major career goal will have to be grounded in basic research methodology. This foundation is most efficiently acquired in a university setting where expert methodologists can provide guidance to the new investigator. We have not attempted to lay out specific course titles because that selection will depend on what is available and should meet the focused needs of the individual faculty member. However, in the implementation plans we do identify generic research methods topics that a faculty member with strong research interests should master.

In determining how to begin to develop new faculty members' research skills, we feel that it is best to let the participant's interest drive the selection of methods, rather than begin with coursework on the different research methodologies. This rationale should help readers understand why activities related to reading the research literature, using a medical library, and conducting an integrated research review are included in the curricula. A prerequisite to all successful research is a thorough knowledge of one's interest area. After this, an overview of different methodologies is appropriate; then curricula should branch out in individual directions.

Several learning principles guided the design of the courses. Basic cognitive competencies were addressed with strategies such as readings and lecture/demonstrations, followed by small group discussion. To accomplish midlevel abilities, homework assignments, in-class assignments, and simulations were added. Highest-level competencies are addressed through the research project and presentation.

Annotated Bibliography

The references below were considered especially important to the content expert in defining and developing this domain. Therefore, they have been annotated, while other cited works have been included only in the Reference section. (For complete citations of these annotations and all the writings mentioned in this domain, turn to the Reference section at the end of this chapter.)

Annotations can be very illuminating to readers for a number of reasons. First, they give readers who are not particularly familiar with the subject matter some important background information—a kind of "Cliff's Notes" to the curriculum content. Second, many of the annotations point to specific chapters or excerpts that may stimulate new ideas for teaching or provide you with "quick-and-dirty" teaching materials. Third, they can help direct whatever further literature searches you may be planning in the area on your own.

Last but not least, the discerning reader will learn much about the content expert's vision, perspective, or philosophic stance regarding his or her subject by reading these deliberately selected annotations. Perhaps even more than the prose in each rationale section, this bibliography may help you to see the subject matter as the content expert saw it and to understand why the domain is structured the way it is.

Content Knowledge

Cooper, H. M. (1984). *The integrative research review: A systematic approach.*

This is an excellent introduction to the science and art of conducting systematic research reviews. The author provides many practical examples, figures, and checklists that are easy to follow. Four stages for conducting a research review are examined in detail: problem formation; data collection; data evaluation analyses, and interpretation and presentation. The chapter on data evaluation is a particularly important one. The author fully describes the "quantitative revolution" in research reviews— a methodology based on statistical techniques that measures strengths of relationship and effect size from multiple independent studies.

Gehlbach, S. H. (1988). *Interpreting the medical literature: A clinician's guide.*

This book presents a logical approach to understanding research literature for the primary care physician. Numerous examples from clinical research are included, which makes it easier to read than the average text. The organization of the book parallels the sequence of a research article and in so doing gives readers the necessary tools to evaluate the primary components of a research study. The chapters on statistical significance, predictive values, and risk are particularly helpful.

Kuhn, T. (1964). *The structure of scientific revolutions.*

An excellent discussion of how science develops and how scientific paradigms are accepted and rejected throughout time. Kuhn takes a historical perspective by charting the nature of "normal science" and then describes how scientific discoveries occur through anomalies and crises. The final chapters address the necessity of scientific revolutions and the progress made by them. This book works well for a seminar on the history or philosophy of science. A classic that any serious researcher should read.

Light, R. J., & Pillemer, D. B. (1984). *Summing up: The science of reviewing research.*

This book offers six chapters that focus on basic steps in conducting a research review. Sample chapter titles include: "Organizing a Reviewing Strategy"; "Quantitative Procedures"; "Numbers and Narrative"; "What We Have Learned"; and "Checklist for Evaluating Reviews." A framework is presented that helps the novice organize the literature and synthesize the sometimes contradictory results. Examples and a 10-question checklist are provided.

This is a very practical book for both beginning and experienced researchers, although some statistical background is assumed. Like Cooper, the authors propose a qualitative method for comparing multiple studies, which then allows the reviewer to make summary statements about the data sets from different studies.

Riegelman, R. K. (1981). *Studying a study and testing a test: How to read the medical literature.*

The aim of this book is to provide a step-by-step approach to literature review. Assuming that the reader has had no prior training in statistics or epidemiology, the author presents four self-contained units that explain how to evaluate studies, tests, rates, and statistics found in journal articles. The four units are: "Studying a Study," "Testing a Test," "Rating a Rate," and "Selecting a Statistic." The book is easy to read and includes very useful flaw-catching exercises.

Sackett, D. L., Haynes, R. B., & Tugwell, P. (1985). *Clinical epidemiology: A basic science for clinical medicine.*

Part III of this book is entitled "Keeping Up to Date." In it the authors provide a helpful service to the practicing physician by describing a procedure for reviewing and evaluating one's own clinical performance. Also in this section are chapters entitled: "How to Use a Library"; and "Getting the Most from Continuing Education." The chapter on reading a clinical journal is a good summary of the guides that have appeared in the Canadian Medical Association Journal in the past.

Methodological Skills

Bailer, J. C., & Mosteller, F. (1986). *Medical uses of statistics.*

Another "second-level" book on statistics, "This book surveys the state-of-the-art statistical applications in clinical research and illustrates good and poor uses of methods" (Introduction). Thirteen of the 20 chapters were originally published in the *New England Journal of Medicine* between 1983 and 1985. While this text draws heavily on clinical examples, there are no exercises, unfortunately, to facilitate the reader's exploration of good and poor uses of methods.

Colton, T. (1982). *Statistics in medicine.*

This book examines statistical principles from the view of the research consumer, the reader. Part I introduces basic concepts, definitions, and principles of descriptive statistics and probability. Part II builds a foundation for understanding statistical inference and drawing conclusions about populations based on data from samples. These chapters cover the most frequently used statistical tests encountered in the general medical literature. Part III discusses the use of statistics in medical research and contains chapters on clinical trials and medical surveys, then identifies common pitfalls to drawing conclusions from medical research.

Feinstein, A. R. (1977). *Clinical biostatistics.*

This book is based upon nearly 40 journal essays the author has written for *Clinical Pharmacology and Therapeutics*. Section one is an introduction to Feinstein's concept of the "architecture" of cohort research. Section two is a continuation of this theme that also includes sampling, bias, and control issues as they relate to research. Section three focuses on measurement problems. Section four addresses mathematical mystiques and statistical strategies and common pitfalls in reasoning with statistics. Finally, section five focuses on analytic strategies for multiple variables. The book is informative and enjoyable but presumes some knowledge of biostatistics.

Godfrey, K. (1985). *Comparing the means of several groups.*

Based upon her observation that researchers frequently employ statistical methods incorrectly when comparing the means of several groups, Godfrey offers a very clear, fundamental explanation as to why multiple *t*-tests should not be used. Using examples from original articles in the *New England Journal of Medicine*, she discusses more appropriate analyses, such as analysis of variance and multiple comparison techniques.

Godfrey, K. (1985). Simple linear regression in medical research.

This excellent article introduces linear regression analysis to the physician researcher. First, it overviews a method for fitting a straight line to data; the method is described (and applied) in reference to 36 original articles from the *New England Journal of Medicine*. Second, the author stresses that readers and researchers must also attend to residuals as an important aspect of regression analysis. Finally, there is a discussion of popular statistical packages that provide regression analysis and data plots.

Henry, R. C., Massa, M. D., & Ogle, K. S. (1985). *Planning a research study.*

This packaged workshop and workbook materials are designed to teach new researchers how to prepare a research plan for their first study. The exercises engage participants in developing hypotheses and operational definitions, preparing a research design, and drawing up a timeline and flow chart for research activities. Participants also define outcome measures and establish procedures for data collection using those measures.

Henry, R. C., & Zivick, J. D. (1986). *Principles of survey research.*

An introduction to survey research that explains 10 basic principles to consider when designing surveys. This article also includes an item-writing checklist for evaluating questionnaire items. The emphasis is on mailed questionnaires and includes discussion of sample size, response rates, and survey format.

Hulley, S. B., & Cummings, S. R. (Eds.). (1988). *Designing Clinical Research.*

Based upon their experience in teaching clinical research methods the authors write an excellent guide to the steps one takes in developing and implementing a clinical research study. The practical examples serve as useful models for the beginning researcher.

Kelsey, J. L., Thompson, W. D., & Evans, A. S. (1986). *Methods in observational epidemiology.*

Consider this book a good companion to an introductory textbook on epidemiology or as a resource for planning epidemiologic research. The first three chapters review elementary epidemiologic and biostatistical concepts and methods usually covered in introductory courses. The remaining chapters describe commonly used study designs (e.g., prospective and retrospective cohort studies, cross-sectional and case control studies). Finally, issues related to measurement, error, and sample size are addressed in detail. There are study exercises but no answers to the questions.

Kleinbaum, D. G., Kupper, L. L., & Morgenstern, H. (1982). *Epidemiologic research.*

This text discusses the principles, concepts, and methods involved in the planning, analysis, and interpretation of epidemiologic research. The author's purpose is to synthesize methodologic practice and thought. Specifically, the text emphasizes quantitative and statistical issues. Nearly 100 pages are devoted to a most helpful discussion of the validity of epidemiologic research. For the more advanced reader.

Koran, L. M. (1973). *The reliability of clinical methods, data and judgments.*

A useful article that addresses the reliability of diagnoses, laboratory tests, and clinical observations.

Levy, R. S., & Lemeshow, S. (1980). *Sampling for health professionals.*

Written for researchers who are experienced in survey design, this text includes many applied techniques and practical examples. The emphasis of the book is on sample design, and it describes sampling techniques ranging from simple to cluster, stratified, and stage sampling. The authors also include chapters on response, data collection forms, and interpretation of data for report writing. Practice exercises and a solutions manual are available.

Marks, R. G. (1982). *Analyzing research data. The basics of biomedical research methodology.*

This book teaches fundamental statistical techniques used in analyzing and evaluating clinical data. Emphasis is on selection of the appropri-

ate statistical analysis and interpretation of data from computer printouts. While not as comprehensive as some texts, it does focus on essential
techniques such as the *t-* and *Z*-tests, ANOVA, nonparametric techniques, discriminant analysis, and time series. This and Marks' other
book (see below) assume no previous knowledge of statistics and design
issues.

Marks, R. G. (1982). *Designing a research project: The basics of
biomedical research methodology.*

This book teaches the basic concepts of research design through a step-
by-step guide. It explains how to determine project objectives, decide
which type of data to collect, and design a data collection form. Two
very practical chapters describe how to determine the proper sample
size for the study.

Mausner, J. S., & Kramer, S. (1985). *Epidemiology: An introductory text.*

The second edition of this introductory text was published 2 years after
the death of the first author. It remains an easy-to-read, well-organized
introduction to the principles of epidemiology. Its 13 chapters describe
a number of basic concepts including multiple causation of disease, rates,
ratios and proportions, screening, and types of analytic studies.

Niemi, R. G., & Sullivan, J. L. (Eds.). *Quantitative applications
in the social sciences.*

Although written for social scientists, these are practical, inexpensive
monographs that are designed to improve the methodological skills of
all researchers. There are over 60 papers in this series that focus on
a variety of research topics for the beginning and advanced researcher.
The papers are clearly written and are as useful for the primary care
researcher as they are for the social scientist. A sampling of titles: "Tests
of significance," "Analysis of Variance," "Analysis of Nominal and Ordinal
Data," "Factor Analysis," "Measures of Association," "Survey Sampling."
For a complete listing of titles and descriptions write the publisher: Sage
Publications, P.O. Box 5024, Beverly Hills, California 90210, (312)
274-8003.

Nunnally, J. C. (1984). *Psychometric theory.*

This comprehensive text on scientific measurement will make a substantial contribution to any researcher's library. The book addresses numerous important issues in measurement theory such as the internal structure of measures, validity, construction of tests and measures, factor analytic techniques, and multidimensional scaling.

O'Brien, P. C., & Shampo, M. A. (1981). *Statistics for clinicians.*

A reprint series available from *The Mayo Clinical Proceedings*. A most practical overview of descriptive and inferential statistical techniques used in clinical research. The writing is nontechnical and very appropriate for the beginning researcher. In all there are 12 papers that briefly address the following topics in statistics: descriptive statistics; graphic displays; estimation from samples; one- and two-sample t-tests; regression; chi-square and the relative deviate test; evaluating diagnostic procedures; normal values; survivorship studies and sequential methods.

Schefler, W. C. (1984). *Statistics for health professionals.*

A good introduction to statistics that does not assume any mathematics beyond high school algebra. The emphasis is placed on applied statistics as a set of principles and a way of thinking rather than a series of exercises in mathematics. The chapter on probability is especially well written in that it incorporates many examples from specific diseases that are common to clinical medicine. Similar to other introductory textbooks, the author includes chapters on comparing means, proportions, regression analysis, correlations, and analysis of covariance. The new researcher may find this to be one of the most readable texts on statistics.

Velleman, P. F., & Hoaglin, D. C. (1981). *Applications, basics and computing of exploratory data analysis.*

Exploratory data analysis (EDA) represents a new tradition in statistics popularized by Princeton statistics Professor John W. Tukey in his 1977 book *Exploratory Data Analysis*. This practical philosophy of data analysis does not use the traditional hypothesis-driven analysis techniques, rather it uses EDA and proceeds much in the way a detective might solve a mystery. The behavior and nature of data are examined for patterns and trends, and from these observations statistical analyses are selected. The EDA approach to statistics is an interactive and dynamic one that takes advantage of computer graphics programs. Velleman is a former student of Tukey who has rendered EDA both practical and fun to new researchers through a new software program for the Macintosh computer (Data Desk Professional II, Odesta Corp., Northbrook, IL). As the name implies, this book provides the ABCs of how to incorporate EDA into understanding one's own data sets.

Young, M. J., Bresnitz, E. A., & Strom, B. L. (1983). *Sample size nomogram for interpreting negative clinical studies.*

The big question for many researchers is, "How many subjects do I need?" This brief article provides a useful strategy for using a nomogram to interpret negative studies and also to determine sample size for projected studies. A practical example is included for readers to apply the nomogram to a real research situation.

Management Skills

Berg, A. O., Gordon, M. J., & Cherkin, D. C. (1986). *Practice based research in family medicine.*

A monograph published by the American Academy of Family Physicians to assist practitioners in their preparation for research. Use it as a resource handbook rather than a text or how-to manual on research. The monograph includes chapters on focusing a study question, locating the literature, obtaining funding, and data collection. It also includes Gordon's (1978) *Research Workbook*, which is a helpful guide in research planning.

McGaghie, W. C., & Frey, J. J. (1986). *Handbook for the academic physician.*

This very handy and informative book has six chapters that focus on clinical research. Topics range from a discussion of the role of research in primary care medicine to the specifics of data management. This book is well-suited for the beginning researcher who needs guidance in identifying funding resources and in constructing a plan for managing the study.

References

Ahlgren, A. (1983). *Practical data analysis with SPSS* (package of 12 videotapes for using and interpreting SPSS). Minneapolis: University of Minnesota, Media Distribution.

Alguire, P., Henry, R., Massa, M., & Lienhart, K. (1986). *Power reading: Critical appraisal of the medical literature.* East Lansing, MI: Michigan State University, Office of Medical Education Research and Development.

Bailer, J. C., & Mosteller, F. (1986). *Medical uses of statistics.* Waltham, MA: New England Journal of Medicine Books.

Berg, A. O., Gordon, M. J., & Cherkin, D. C. (1986). *Practice based research in family medicine,* Kansas City, MO: American Academy of Family Physicians.

Bland, C. J., & Schmitz, C. C. (1986). Characteristics of the successful researcher and implications for faculty development. *Journal of Medical Education, 61,* 22–31.

Brown, G. W. (1980). Regression and clinical research. *American Journal of Diseases of Children, 134,* 549–552.

Brown, G. W. (1981). Bayes' formula: Conditional probability and clinical medicine. *American Journal of Diseases of Children, 135,* 1125–1129.

Brown, G. W. (1982). Standard deviation, standard error: Which "standard" should we use? *American Journal of Diseases of Children, 136,* 937–941.

Brown, G. W. (1983). Errors, types I and II. *American Journal of Diseases of Children, 137,* 586–591.

Brown, G. W. (1984). Discriminant analysis. *American Journal of Diseases of Children, 138,* 395–400.

Brown, G. W. (1985a). Counts, scales and scores. *American Journal of Diseases of Children, 139,* 147–151.

Brown, G. W. (1985b). Statistics and the medical journal [Editorial]. *American Journal of Diseases of Children, 139,* 226–228.

Brown, G. W., (1985c). 2 × 2 tables. *American Journal of Diseases of Children, 139,* 410–416.

Brown, G. W., & Hayden, G. F. (1985). Nonparametric methods: Clinical applications. *Clinical Pediatrics, 24*(9), 490–498.

Bulpitt, C. J. (1987). Confidence intervals. *Lancet, 1,* 494–496.

Butterfield, H. (1960). *The origins of modern science.* New York: Macmillan.

Colton, T. (1982). *Statistics in medicine.* Boston: Little, Brown.

Cooper, H. M. (1984). *The integrative research review: A systematic approach.* Beverly Hills, CA: Sage Publications.

Cuddy, P. G., Elenbaas, R. M., & Elenbaas, J. K. (1983). Evaluating the medical literature, Part I: Abstract, introduction, methods. *Annals of Emergency Medicine, 12,* 549–555.

Elenbaas, J. K., Cuddy, P. G., & Elenbaas, R. M. (1983). Evaluating the medical literature, Part III: Results and discussion. *Annals of Emergency Medicine, 12,* 610–620.

Elenbaas, R. M., Elenbaas, J. K., & Cuddy, P. G. (1983). Evaluating the medical literature, Part II: Statistical analysis. *Annals of Emergency Medicine, 12,* 679–686.

Feinstein, A. R. (1977). *Clinical biostatistics.* St. Louis: C. V. Mosby.

Fletcher, R. H., Fletcher, S. W., & Wagner, E. H. (1988). *Clinical epidemiology: The essentials* (2nd ed.). Baltimore: Williams & Wilkins.

The Foundation Center. (1979). *The Foundation Directory* (7th ed.). New York: Author.

Gehlbach, S. H. (1988). *Interpreting the medical literature: A clinician's guide* (2nd ed.). Lexington, MA: D.C. Heath.

Geyman, J. P. (1978). On the developing research base in family practice. *Journal of Family Practice, 7*(1), 51–52.

Geyman, J. P. (1980). Health services research: A crucial and underfunded need. *Journal of Family Practice, 11*(2), 195–196.

Geyman, J. P., & Berg, A. O. (1984). 1974–1983: Analysis of an evolving literature base. *Journal of Family Practice, 18*(1), 47–51.

Godfrey, K. (1985a). Comparing the means of several groups. *New England Journal of Medicine, 313,* 1450–1456.

Godfrey, K. (1985b). Simple linear regression in medical research. *New England Journal of Medicine, 313,* 1629–1636.

Goldman, L., Mushlin, A. I., & Lee, K. L. (1986, July–August). Using medical data bases for clinical research. *Journal of General Internal Medicine, 1* (4 Suppl.), S25–S30.

Gordon, M. J. (1978). Research traditions available to family medicine. *Journal of Family Practice, 7,* 59–66.

Green, L. A., Wood, M., Becker, L., Farley, E. S. Jr., Freeman, W. L., Froom, J., Hames, C., Niebauer, L. G., Rosser, W. W., & Seifert, M. (1984). The ambulatory sentinel practice network: Purpose, methods and policies. *Journal of Family Practice, 18*(2), 275–280.

Guba, E. G. (1978). *Toward a methodology of naturalistic inquiry in educational evaluation* (Evaluation Monograph No. 8). Los Angeles: University of California Center for the Study of Evaluation.

Guilford, J. P. (1975). *Psychometric methods* (3rd ed.). New York: McGraw-Hill.

Hall, M. (1977). *Developing skills in proposal writing* (2nd ed.). Portland, OR: Continuing Education Publications.

Hayden, G. F., Kramer, M. S., & Horowitz, R. I. (1982). The case-control study. *Journal of the American Medical Association, 247,* 326–331.

Henry, R. C., Massa, M. D., & Ogle, K. S. (1985). *Planning a research study.* East Lansing, MI: Michigan State University, Office of Medical Education Research and Development.

Henry, R. C., & Zivick, J. D. (1986). Principles of survey research. *Family Practice Research Journal, 5,* 145–153.

Hulley, S. B., & Cummings, S. R. (Eds.). (1988). *Designing Clinical Research,* Baltimore, MD: Williams & Wilkins.

Huth, E. J. (1986). The primary care research environment. *Journal of General Internal Medicine, 1* (Suppl.), 55–57.

Kelsey, J. L., Thompson, W. D., & Evans, A. S. (1986). *Methods in observational epidemiology.* New York: Oxford University Press.

Kleinbaum, D. G., Kupper, L. L., & Morgenstern, H. (1982). *Epidemiologic research.* Belmont, CA: Wadsworth.

Koran, L. M. (1973). The reliability of clinical methods, data and judgments. *New England Journal of Medicine, 293,* 642–646.

Kramer, M. S., & Feinstein, A. R. (1981). Clinical biostatistics: The biostatistics of concordance. *Clinical Pharmacology and Therapy, 29,* 111–123.

Kramer, H. C., & Thierman, S. (1987). *How many subjects? Statistical power analysis in research.* Newburg Park, CA: Sage Publications.

Krathwohl, D. R. (1966). *How to prepare a research proposal.* Syracuse, NY: Syracuse University Bookstore.

Kuhn, T. (1964). *The structure of scientific revolutions.* Chicago: University of Chicago Press.

Levy, R. S., & Lemeshow, S. (1980). *Sampling for health professionals.* Belmont, CA: Wadsworth.

Light, R. J., & Pillemer, D. B. (1984). *Summing up: The science of reviewing research.* Cambridge, MA: Harvard University Press.

Locke, L. F., Spirduso, W. W., & Silverman, S. J. (1987). *Proposals that work.* Newburg Park, CA: Sage Publications.

Marcus, A. C., & Crane, L. A. (1986). Telephone surveys in public health research. *Medical Care, 24*(2), 97–112.

Marks, R. G. (1982a). *Analyzing research data: The basics of biomedical research methodology.* Belmont, CA: Wadsworth.

Marks, R. G. (1982b). *Designing a research project: The basics of biomedical research methodology.* Belmont, CA: Wadsworth.

Masterman, L. E. (1978). *The applicant's guide to successful grantsmanship.* Cape Girardeau, MO: Keene Publications.

Mausner, J. S., & Kramer, S. (1985). *Epidemiology: An introductory text.* Philadelphia, PA: W. B. Saunders.

McGaghie, W. C., & Frey, J. J. (1986). *Handbook for the academic physician.* New York: Springer-Verlag.

McGraw-Hill. (1978). *McGraw-Hill's guide to health grants and contracts.* Washington, DC: Author.

Moses, L. E. (1985). Statistical concepts fundamental to investigations. *New England Journal of Medicine, 312*(14), 890–897.

National Library of Medicine. (1985). *The basics of searching MEDLINE: A guide for the health professional.* Bethesda, MD: Author.

Niemi, R. G., & Sullivan, J. L. (Eds.). (1976). *Quantitative applications in the social sciences.* Newburg Park, CA: Sage Publications.

Norman, G. R., & Streiner, D. L. (1986). *PDQ statistics.* Toronto: B. C. Decker.

Nunnally, J. C. (1984). *Psychometric theory* (3rd ed.). New York: McGraw-Hill.

O'Brien, P. C., & Shampo, M. A. (1981). Statistics for clinicians [Special Series]. *Mayo Clinical Proceedings, 56,* 45–61.

Patton, M. W. (1975). Alternative evaluation research paradigm. *North Dakota*

Study Group on Evaluation Monograph Series. Grand Forks, ND: University of North Dakota.

Perkoff, G. T. (1981). Research in family medicine: Classification, direction and costs. *Journal of Family Practice, 13*(4), 553–562.

Platt, J. R. (1964). Strong inference. *Science, 146,* 347–353.

Riegelman, R. K. (1981). *Studying a study and testing a test: How to read the medical literature.* Boston: Little, Brown.

Sackett, D. L., Hanes, R. B., & Tugwell, P. (1985). *Clinical epidemiology: A basic science for clinical medicine.* Boston: Little, Brown.

Schefler, W. C. (1984). *Statistics for health professionals.* Reading, MA: Addison-Wesley.

True, J. A. (1983). *Finding out: Conducting and evaluating social research.* Belmont, CA: Wadsworth Pub. Co.

U.S. Department of Health and Human Services. (1986). *NIH guide for grants and contracts* (Vol. 15, No. 2). Bethesda, MD: Author.

U.S. Government Printing Office. (1985). *Update to the catalog of federal domestic assistance.* Washington, DC: Author.

Velleman, P. F., & Hoaglin, D. C. (1981). *Applications, basics and computing of exploratory data analysis.* Boston: Duxbury Press.

Washington report on medicine and health (Vol. 39, No. 34). Washington, DC: McGraw-Hill.

Young, M. J., Bresnitz, E. A., & Strom, B. L. (1983). Sample size nomogram for interpreting negative clinical studies. *Annals of Internal Medicine, 99*(2), 248–253.

CHAPTER **6**

Written Communication Domain

Introduction to the Domain

Writing is, for most, laborious and slow. The mind travels faster than the pen; consequently, writing becomes a question of learning to make occasional wing shots, bringing down the bird of thought as it flashes by. A writer is a gunner, sometimes waiting in his blind for something to come in, sometimes roaming the countryside to scare something up. Like other gunners, he must cultivate patience; he may have to work many covers to bring down one partridge.

—E. B. White (Strunk & White, 1979, p. 69)

The ability to write well is a valued asset in academic medicine, largely because it leads to valued products such as training or research grants, scholarly publications, course materials, administrative documents, and the like. These and other forms of writing demand no small range of skills. In fact, at least one author has called the research article a "cunningly contrived piece of rhetoric" (Ziman, 1969). Others (they shall remain nameless) have decreed the grant application an invention of the devil. Such epithets are deserved. Academic writing requires mastery of basic skills (e.g., how to write complete sentences with nouns and verbs in the active voice) as well as specialized and complex writing strategies (e.g., how to write for a particular journal, articulate abstract concepts, synthesize complex data, or engender confidence). To be successful, a writer *does* need to cultivate the patience of a gunner.

Definition of the Written Communication Domain

The origin of these important skills can be traced to two categories of nonfiction prose in the lineage of written English: *technical writing* (as in business, government, education, and other professions), and *scholarly writing* (for the academic disciplines, especially in science and medicine). Both technical and scholarly writing developed out of the oral tradition and the principles of rhetoric, as they were conceived in ancient Greece and Rome and shaped over the centuries by language scholars, literary critics, great literary masters, and the habits of literate people (see Figure 6.1 below).

The definition of rhetoric has changed little since Aristotle's day, when it signified "the art of communication" (Corbett, 1977). although its practice expanded in the eighteenth century to include written forms of expression as well as speech-making. In contrast to creative writing, the rhetoric of communication is concerned with the logical presentation of ideas and critical analyses of fact. To Aristotle, the original empiricist, "rhetoric strengthened truth and justice" (Young, 1979). Today's English texts and rhetoric handbooks address diction, grammar, composition, style, and other matters related to writing expository prose—whether that prose ultimately results in narration, instruction, persuasion, entertainment, or truth and justice.

Several authorities in rhetoric and scholarly writing served as references and resources for the competencies and teaching strategies for this domain. Strunk and White (1979) and the University of Chicago Press (1969) are probably the two most widely cited sources on style and usage, and they provided this domain with much of its foundation. Barzun (1975), Corbett (1977), Altick (1969), and Tichy (1966) cover the principles of rhetoric. Dirckx (1977), Day (1979), Huth (1982), and King (1978) relate practical information very well in their manuals on medical and scientific writing. Fielden (1964, 1982) and others (STFM Task Force on Professional Communication Skills, 1984) discuss the "shoulds" of administrative writing. In addition to these texts by master writers, editors, and teachers, the research literature on writing (especially the cognitive processes of writing) was consulted (Flower & Hayes, 1981; Hayes & Flower, 1986; Scardamalia & Bereiter, 1986). Additional background on the research on readability and the writing process is provided by McLaughlin (1969) and Boice and Ferdinand (1984). Woodford (1967) and Ziman (1969) offer interesting perspectives on critical thinking and the role of scientific communication.

In all of these texts, variations on the traditional themes of rhetoric repeat themselves: the audience is important; the writing process is iterative and requires cycles of organization and refinement;

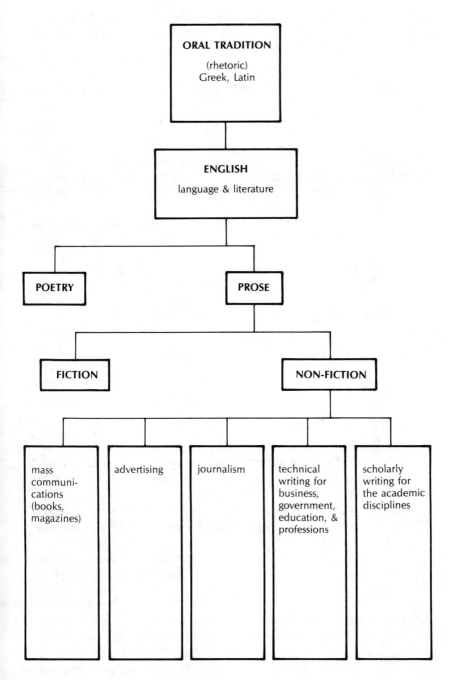

FIGURE 6.1 Origin of written communication skills.

the conventions of format and medium need to be respected. In the final analysis, expressive language is that which is simple, direct, and "makes sense."

Rational for Including Written Communication in the Curriculum

The ability to write well (indeed, to write at all) has long been considered "the mark of an educated man" (Altick, 1969). A more useful rationale for writing well, however, comes from E. B. White (Strunk & White, 1979), who admonishes us to write clearly out of consideration for our readers. Others cite the Golden Rule: "Write unto others as you would have them write unto you."

When constructing this curriculum we targeted written instead of oral communication skills for several reasons:

1. In 1981, a professional organization serving the discipline of family medicine surveyed its members about desired areas for potential faculty development (Society for Teachers of Family Medicine Task Force on Professional Communication, 1984). Their questionnaire included, as options, both written and oral communication. Survey results indicated that "the greatest challenge lay in the area of written communication skills, [and] the needs are not confined to medical articles and book writing, but extend to the full range of academic communication, p. v).

2. Writing is a critical skill used in each of the academic roles (research, teaching, and administration).

3. The mechanics of writing are taught at no other time in medical schools, residency programs, or this curriculum, whereas the Education domain includes a section on oral delivery skills.

4. The risks of being unclear are higher in writing than in speech, the consequences greater (Boice & Ferdinand, 1984; Graves & Hodge, 1979).

5. Promotion in academe depends on quantity and quality of publications, a challenge for writers whatever their degree of experience.

In summary, well-written pieces communicate (inform, educate, inspire, synthesize the literature, move entire committees to action); poorly written ones do not. Moreover, the link between critical thinking and writing ability works both ways (Woodford, 1967); as one works to improve skills in the latter, the former also gains.

How the Domain Has Been Structured

Once established in academic medicine, faculty members may communicate in writing to as many as five different audiences: patients, students, administrators, government and foundation personnel, and colleagues. These audiences typically require a particular format or publication type(s), as displayed in Figure 6.2.

Although faculty may also write letters to colleagues, newsletters for colleagues, or other combinations, they typically work with new publication formats whenever they change audiences. Most faculty writing occurs in the administration and colleague categories.

Although each publication format and each audience require special stylistic considerations, all share a need for similar organizational and technical skills. The competencies in this section reflect, therefore, these across-the-board process skills. (Specific instructions for preparing research articles, student workbooks, or grants, for example, will have to be specified by faculty developers/teachers during coursework or consultation.) The competencies within this domain have been organized according to four skills clusters:

1. Writing for the particular audience
2. Organizing content, the message at hand
3. Writing within the given publication type and format
4. Applying rules of English usage, style, and composition

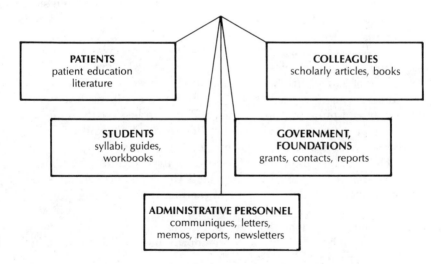

FIGURE 6.2 Audiences and forms of written communication in academic medicine.

Perhaps another way to reduce the sum of knowledge about writing competency to digestible components is to say that to write any of the products for audiences listed above, faculty need to: (1) know the audience, (2) know the content, (3) know the format and structure that house the message, and (4) know basic rules of language and writing technique.

These four areas also express a logical sequence of events within the writing process. After recognizing an occasion or purpose for writing, an author identifies the audience, which immediately shapes (to a small or large degree) the organization and presentation of content. He or she then drafts the message to work within a particular format and its conventions, then revises and edits his or her language to meet standards of usage and style.

The domain of skills could reasonably be broken down in other ways, for example by faculty role (administrator, teacher, researcher), by product (letter, newsletter, manual, proposal), or by content subareas (composition, diction, grammar). To teach the skills of writing, some of these divisions may be desirable. But to analyze the underlying generic abilities and state them as competencies, the schema above seems preferable.

Assumptions Made in Constructing the Domain

Traditionalists may argue that these components fail to emphasize enough the importance of English usage and style. Usage and style do receive considerable attention in terms of time in the suggested curriculum, although they represent only one of the four subareas. It is our feeling, however, that the offenses of nonparallel sentence structure, split infinitives, and dangling participles are less serious than lack of organization, inappropriate language or vocabulary for the audience, or confused thought. Editors can help writers whose grammar and punctuation are rusty. They can less easily remedy a manuscript whose author has not understood the conventions of his medium or identified a critical purpose of writing.

The greatest impediment facing faculty authors who wish to write is lack of momentum: they lack the habit of writing small amounts each day and the habit of reading (with a thoughtful ear) what they, and others, have written. As one teacher was quoted as saying, students and faculty new to writing should be encouraged to develop the habit of "writing things down (but not necessarily 'up' as finished products)" (Young, 1979).

The second impediment facing faculty is lack of a few basic skills for organizing their sentences, their paragraphs, and their content.

Surveys have shown that faculty who publish have no more available time at their disposal than nonpublishers (Boice & Ferdinand, 1984); what they do have is momentum and enough skills to use well the time they have. Learning to write well does take time, and it takes guided practice. It also takes patience and the willingness to incorporate the advice of editors. The challenge to faculty development is to make the opportunities for skill-building and consultation available—and rewarding.

Goals and Competencies

Listed below are suggested goals and competencies in the domain of written communication for academic faculty. This list is comprehensive in the sense that the competencies are not targeted to particular institutions or faculty types. For suggestions on how to pull out relevant competencies for preceptors, non-tenure-track, and tenure-track faculty, see Chapter 2.

These goals and competencies were prepared by the content expert through a process involving literature review, meetings with physician liaisons and advisory committee members, and three surveys. We list them here according to the major subareas of the domain, as identified earlier.

Writing for the Particular Audience

GOAL 18.0: To communicate effectively to different audiences.

No matter what the genre, writing *for* the audience is a cardinal rule that most of us break routinely. Unconsciously, we write for ourselves or people like us. In doing so we bore the readers who already know our message, confuse those who do not, miss opportunities to inform when information is needed, and offend readers who hold different perspectives or consider certain words or topics taboo. Writers who can hear how their message "sounds" to their readers stand a better chance of being understood and valued.

Faculty should be able to:

18.1. Test own methods for knowing one's audience
18.2. Describe both a typical member of the audience and the variety of people that comprise it
18.3. Specify the elements of knowledge and experience the audience has (or does not have) related to the topic

18.4. Determine why the audience may want or need one's information or viewpoints
18.5. List the criteria by which the audience will judge one's written material

Organizing Content, the Message at Hand

GOAL 19.0: To develop process strategies for organizing and drafting written material.

To write is to organize one's thoughts: to gather, scan, select, combine, sequence, edit, and empower pieces of knowledge for a particular audience. In written medical communication, both the process of preparing to write and writing itself depend on organizational skills, which in turn rely on critical thinking and reading skills.

Competencies in this section have been divided into two groups. Together they reflect problems and strategies inherent to the organizing process. The first group applies to material from all publication types, the second to longer pieces only, such as evaluation reports, research articles, student guides, and books.

Faculty should be able to:

19.1. State the primary purpose for writing
19.2. Explain what is new, different, or important about the message or content
19.3. List (or diagram) the primary points of the message and their connections
19.4. Determine the background information (facts, definitions, references) readers need in order to understand the content
19.5. Determine boundaries for the subject: which points or topics get included, which excluded
19.6. Establish who's "talking" (writing), in which tense (past, present, future)

For longer material

19.7. Read with a critical ear to develop or test ideas
19.8. Implement a system for abstracting/documenting literature and other sources of information on their topic
19.9. Develop whatever intrinsic structure the content has and adapt it to the publication format
19.10. Use frameworks for structuring material, such as diagrams and notes, content outlines, minidrafts, etc.

19.11. Schedule a timetable for writing that encourages systematic and frequent writing sessions

19.12. Build in a mechanism for evaluation and revision (e.g., pilot test, second or third readers, editor/proofreader)

Wrting Within the Given Publication Type and Format

GOAL 20.0: To prepare material according to general and specific format guidelines

Theoretically, publication formats evolve to suit the nature of the content, its purpose, and the audience. They also serve (sometimes arbitrarily) stylistic conventions of editors and publishing communities. For example, the Introduction–Methods–Results–Discussion (IMRD) format and passive voice flourish in medical writing because the IMRD formula best reveals the (almost) invariable process steps of a research study, and passive voice constructions suggest (to some readers) scientific detachment. The organizational format has a defensible rationale; the passive voice persists despite changing editorial fashion. In other publication categories, format and style are combined more advantageously. For example, patient education literature often addresses their readers' most predictable needs with a simply worded, direct, question-and-answer format. To assist learning, student guides highlight course objectives and principal concepts and insert practice/feedback sections or summaries at regular intervals.

Using the specific guidelines of a particular publication (e.g., *Journal of the American Medical Association*) and the generic guidelines of a publication type (e.g., teacher guide) makes an author's task easier and requires little skill, once the conventions of each publication type are known. In addition to helping writers frame their material, knowledge of a particular journal's requirements helps faculty determine where it is best to submit their work. The competencies below address general format considerations, journal selection for research articles, and the submission process.

Faculty should be able to:

20.1. Summarize the content requirements each format imposes (Introduction, Methods, Results, Discussion, e.g., MRD) or components of a proposal, parts of a book, elements of a student syllabus, format for business correspondence, etc.

20.2. Access reference materials that detail stylistic and technical conventions of each format (maximum length, reference

style, headings, tables and graphs, photos, other guidelines
for preparing manuscripts)
20.3. Decide when and how to deviate from conventional formats
20.4. Determine how the material will be printed, bound, and delivered before writing*
20.5. Select an appropriate journal for the article*
20.6. Follow protocols for submitting and revising manuscripts*

Applying Rules of Usage, Style, and Composition

GOAL 21.0: To apply rules of English usage, style, and composition.

Having a good command of nouns and verbs helps those of us who write, yet technical knowledge on the level of a prestigious journal editor or Harvard English professor is not necessary to write successfully. Most of the competencies below stress clarity and simplicity of expression rather than intricate elements of speech.

According to Strunk and White (1979), usage refers to rules of grammar, punctuation, capitalization, and the like. The University of Chicago's *Manual of Style* (1969) calls these and similar guidelines "style rules," whereas Tichy (1966) distinguishes between (1) grammar (rules of syntax, punctuation, etc.), (2) composition (arrangement of ideas), and (3) style (richness of language, specificity, eloquence). Dirckx (1977), a most faithful linguist, speaks of usage as Webster's (1973) does: "the way in which words and phrases are actually used (as in a particular form or sense) in a language community" (p. 1279). By this definition, usage applies both to socially acceptable words (for example, "ain't" won't qualify) and acceptable practices (one may now end a sentence with a preposition if the next-to-last word merits the emphasis such placement gives it). To confuse things further, Fielden (1964) uses *style* to mean character or flavor; a "colorful" style, a "warm," "formal," or "scholarly" style are all examples.

The competencies below loosely group current writing conventions and manners in the following way:

Usage   Standard (acceptable) rules of spelling, punctuation, grammar, syntax, capitalization, footnotes, abbreviation, etc.

Style   Preferable writing practices, such as using the active voice, specific and concrete language, brevity. Style also refers to an author's personal manner of speaking.

Composition The arrangement of sentences, paragraphs, and other components such as graphs and tables. Successful "arrangements" in medical writing champion logical thinking, relevance, attention to format, and economy.

Usage is treated minimally here for several reasons. We presume that faculty are, first, minimally competent in grammar and spelling and, second, not in a position to master dozens of detailed rules and exceptions. Also, we place higher premiums on logical expression and a clean writing style. We therefore suggest that developers concentrate on these areas, correcting usage as they go. Often, writers most accomplished in organization and style are also quite particular about the technical details. But for the "occasional" writer just starting out, these details loom large and may all but cause paralysis. Therefore, usage competencies stress the ability to access appropriate reference material and to avoid common errors.

Faculty should be able to:

Usage

21.1. Avoid faulty constructions such as nonparallel sentence structure, dangling participles, misplaced modifiers, run-on sentences, disagreement between subject and verb, and conflicting tenses

21.2. Spell correctly

21.3. Punctuate consistently

21.4. Use words precisely, according to their meaning

21.5. List references according to American Psychological Association or Index Medicus style

21.6. Access resource and reference material for questions on usage

Style

21.7. Write in the active voice

21.8. Choose definite, specific, concrete words

21.9. Avoid sex-biased or culture-biased language

21.10. Decode jargon for the audience

21.11. Eliminate redundancy

21.12. Avoid pompous and overly tentative statements (two sides of the same coin)

21.13. Vary the pattern of sentence structure; vary adjectives, verbs, and nouns

21.14. Allow humor, warmth, or other expressions of feeling to surface when appropriate

21.15. Edit for economy; make "every word tell' (Strunk & White, 1979)

21.16. Vary personal style to suit readers' general background, needs, time frame, and organizational status

Composition

21.17. Make all parts of the text relevant to the central purpose and main ideas

21.18. Work within the given structure of the format and the personal outline

21.19. Provide introductory sentences or paragraphs at the beginning of new and summary sections

21.20. Provide transitions when merging ideas, themes, or facts

21.21. Sequence arguments, concepts, and facts in a logical and persuasive manner

21.22. Provide illustrations (verbal or visual), examples anecdotes, or definitions to suit the audience

21.23. Construct graphs, charts, tables, and figures according to reference guidelines, and base the text on the data as it appears in the visual (not the other way around)

21.24. Proofread for accuracy and completion of design. For example, check that:
- each chapter is listed on the table of contents page
- each reference has a number or citation, and vice versa
- the abstract covers truly principal features of the study
- each "patient question" is answered
- each goal specified has objectives
- each objective specified has instructions
- each enclosure promised has been attached

Courses, Strategies, and Resources

Listed below are suggested courses, strategies, and resources for teaching written communication skills to academic faculty. (To find out which competencies each course or activity addresses, check the numbers listed after each description.) These activities and sources are comprehensive in the sense that they are not keyed to specific faculty types at particular institutions. For guidelines on how to select and combine courses in this (and other) domain(s) for preceptors, non-tenure-track, and tenure-track faculty, see Implementation Models.

401. SUBLIMINAL INSTRUCTION AND MATERIALS CAMPAIGN (Open-ended)

This is not a typical strategy, but a series of reinforcement tactics that a writing consultant can employ given the appropriate materials. The premise of a subliminal instruction and materials campaign is similar to that of advertising: If faculty are exposed frequently to small doses of instruction (i.e., visual messages in the environment), then some learning or absorption will take place. Thus, we have several kinds of tactics to increase faculty's sensitivity to the English language:

1. Daily Maxims may be posted over the coffee area or other place of gathering. Famous errors, principles of English usage, rules of thumb, witty examples, and so forth, may be collected (see Suggested Resource Materials below) and displayed on small signs or posters.
2. Tip Sheets are one-page handouts that may be circulated weekly or monthly in department newsletters; kept on file by an editor and disseminated upon request; posted in secretarial areas; used as reference materials in a common library space; and handed out as instructional material during various faculty development seminars. The content of tip sheets covers a potentially wide range of technical information that is a nuisance to look up yet handy to have on hand, such as:
   • format for references (Index Medicus and American Psychological Association)
   • short reminders (rules) on usage (e.g., when to use commas, semicolons, and colons)
   • lists of frequently misspelled medical terms and other words
   • ten examples of how to rewrite passive voice sentence constructions in the active voice
   • ways to avoid sex-biased language
   • editorial guidelines of selected journals
   • selected biographies

3. Graffiti Boards invite passersby to identify grammatical errors, to rewrite jargon, or to edit interestingly flawed sentences or quotes. Each day a new sentence is written on a centrally located blackboard or easel pad and faculty list corrections or responses below the origi-

nal sentence. Revisions may be anonymous or not, but they should remain on the board all day so various graffiti writers can compare their corrections.

Content for daily maxims, tip sheets, and graffiti boards should be liberally seasoned with medical examples, terms, and contexts. If prepared with a dash of good humor, they can make the routine exposure to correct English (and the style rules for same) easier to digest.

Competencies: 20.1–20.6, 21.1–21.23.

Suggested Resource Material

For complete citations, see the Reference section at the end of this chapter. Also check the Annotated Bibliography for fuller descriptions of some materials.

Barzun, J. (1975). *Simple and direct: A rhetoric for writers.* Lots of good, short exercises and examples, some original, some familiar.

Dirckx, J. H. (1977). *Dx and Rx: A physician's guide to medical writing.* Has commonly misspelled medical words on page 56 and lots of other excerptable matter.

Gordon, K. E. (1983). *The well-tempered sentence: A punctuation handbook for the innocent, the eager, and the doomed.* 100 pages of delightful, one-line sentences illustrating the dos and don'ts of punctuation.

Gordon, I. E. (1984). *The transitive vampire: A handbook of grammar for the innocent, the eager, and the doomed.* As with Gordon's other handbook, this contains page after page of wacky examples, all technically correct.

Graves, R., & Hodge, A. (1979). *The reader over your shoulder: A handbook for writers of English prose.* See their 42 principles of prose, plus examples.

International Committee of Medical Journal Editors. (1982). Uniform requirements for manuscripts submitted to biomedical journals. The consensus of 150 journals from around the world on standards of manuscript preparation, use of abbreviations and symbols, common terms and units of measurements, prior or duplicate publication policies, and other requirements.

King, L. (1978). *Why not say it clearly?* Grammar rules are stated in the chapter entitled "Five Treacherous Servants."

Strunk, W., & White, E. B. (1979). *The elements of style.* The entire book is built around short statements illustrating the principles of writing. The examples are superb, but subtle, not as entertaining as Gordon's.

University of Chicago. (1982). *A manual of style.* Literally hundreds of examples on usage.

402. ONGOING CONSULTATION (Open-ended)

Ongoing consultation with a department or external writing consultant (sometimes known as an author's editor) is a strategy filled with potential learning opportunities. Although the occasion prompting consultations will most likely be the critique of a manuscript, other products (such as grants, syllabi, or newsletter) could certainly benefit from an editor's review. Small pieces, such as the book review, letter-to-the-editor, and newsletter column, could also be used as preliminary writing exercises leading up to longer articles.

A whole range of objectives may be met during individual consults, such as how to write for a particular audience, assemble materials into a draft, develop a systematic approach to writing, improve usage and style, and appreciate the role of published research in a scholarly community. Meeting with the writing consultant should be considered part of every fellowship or faculty development experience.

In working with faculty writing, consultants may take on several roles. They can:

1. Serve as thinking partners; help faculty focus on what they wish to say.
2. Advise them on literature review strategies, on note-taking during the research process, on building mini-summaries and outlines to support the first draft.
3. React to first and second drafts with substantive comments on content, composition, and format guidelines.
4. Teach faculty about their own writing patterns and help them learn new ones, if necessary.
5. Copyedit and proofread manuscripts.
6. Direct faculty to potential publishers and guide them through the submission process.
7. Review with faculty a journal editor's critique of a returned manuscript.
8. Guide their reading habits by suggesting articles and nonmedical literature to read.

Competencies: All

Suggested Resource Material

Many of the references from the Annotated Bibliography or Reference section are applicable here. Particularly relevant are:

Altick, R. D. (1969). *Preface to critical reading.* Specific writing exercises are in chapters on denotation, connotation, diction, determinants of tone, sentences and paragraphs, and patterns of clear thinking.

Boice, R., & Ferdinand, J. (1984). *Why academicians don't write.* Wonderful, extensive bibliography and insight on writing difficulties.

Corbett, E. P. J. (1977). *The little rhetoric handbook.* See Chapter 5 for sentence patterns and subordination.

Rico, G., & Claggett, M. F. (1980). *Balancing the hemispheres: Brain research and the teaching of writing.* Offers clues to teaching students how to approach writing in a nonlinear fashion. Exercises in imaging, diagramming gestalts, then developing sentences are offered.

Waddell, M. L., Esch, R. M., & Walker, R. R. (1972). *The art of styling sentences: Twenty patterns to success.* Offers good examples for practicing variations in sentence structure.

Woodford, F. P. (1968). *Scientific writing for graduate students: A manual on the teaching of scientific writing.* Excellent source for the writing consultant on all points.

403. GRANT-WRITING WORKSHOP (Two full, consecutive days)

A collaborative workshop, co-designed and taught by a grant coordinator (or experienced administrator) and a writing consultant. In 2 days participants learn who the funding sources are and how to identify appropriate ones for training and research grants. In addition, participants learn the basic, generic components of a grant application and experience a mock grant review process.

During the first day, resources for identifying funds are discussed. Actual resource documents (e.g., foundation directories, printout from Sponsored Projects Network Computer runs) are reviewed and people contacts identified. Then, three essential sets of criteria for successful applications are reviewed in a lecture-discussion format. Criteria include the:

1. Minimum requirements concerning time deadlines, formats for packaging, required components of information, appropriate documentation, etc.
2. Features of overall high quality, as seen in material that is consistently logical and clear in its writing, sufficiently detailed and complete in its presentation, and original in concept.

3. Persuasiveness of its rationale section. Here the evidence of need and strength of planning must be presented in a most compelling fashion; arguments should be backed by scholarly evidence and convey the writer's knowledge and expertise.

On the second day, excerpts from actual grant applications are reviewed along with classic samples of rhetorical argument, highlighting the characteristics of persuasive discourse. The typical National Institutes of Health and Health and Human Services grant review processes are then described, and participants proceed with a mock review.

Materials such as vocabulary lists that define key terms, lists of funding agencies, FacSheets from the Bureau of Health Professions, and other helpful hints may be obtained from the sources listed below.

Competencies: 18.1–18.5, 19.1–19.12, 20.1–20.3.

Suggested Resource Material

Bland, C. J. (1987). *Grant-getting: A workshop for the Society of Teachers of Family Medicine.* (Personal teaching materials.)
Bland, C. J., & Moo-Dodge, M. (1984). Grant-getting. In R. B. Taylor & K. A. Munning (Eds.), *Written communication in family medicine.*
DeBakey, L. (1977, July/August). *The persuasive proposal.*
Handouts, videotapes, and packaged materials are available from the Office of Medical Education, Research, and Development, Michigan State University. (Contact William Anderson, Ph.D., 3000 Sunderland, Michigan State University, East Lansing, MI 48910.)
Hennessey, J. L. (1977, July/August). *The unpersuasive proposal.*
Kurzig, C. M. (1980). *Foundation fundamentals: A guide for grant seekers.*
Reif-Leher, L. (1982). *Writing a successful grant application.*
White, V. P. (1975). *Grants: How to find out about them and what to do next.*

404. PREPARING A SCHOLARLY ARTICLE (Two 3-hour sessions, 1 week apart)

Lecture–discussion in tandem with a research consultant. This strategy is designed for the beginning-level faculty author, with the option of inviting experienced authors to attend the more advanced second session.

Session 1 focuses on the basic structure of a scholarly article and the submission process. Topics to cover include choosing an appropriate journal, the IMRD format, and preparing the manuscript. Instructors should explain the link between the IMRD format and the research process; should show how design and data collection activities can be documented (described, tallied) while the research is under way; should demonstrate how the first draft of an article can be based on these field notes and observations. Competencies listed under the areas of audience, organizing the message at hand, and format are most applicable here. At the end of the session, participants should be given two articles to take home, read, and critique before the next week's class.

In Session 2, instructors first review any questions participants had with the topics introduced previously, then go on to critique the two articles. The articles should be clearly different in terms of quality—one first-rate, and the other third-rate. The emphasis here would be on critical analysis of the texts: how well the authors conceptualized their research question, summarized the literature, formulated a research design, presented the results, discussed their findings, and expressed themselves in language. Additional articles (or sections thereof) should be brought along so other points of comparison can be discussed if time permits.

When appropriate, examples of "fuzzy thinking" coexisting with "fuzzy writing" should be highlighted. Similarly, evidence of how clear statements (i.e., those with concrete words, recognizable nouns, verbs in the active voice) can reveal clear thinking should be identified.

Tip sheets and other specifically prepared handouts to distribute include: author's guidelines on journal style; steps in preparing a manuscript; cover letters to journal editors; description of IMRD components; and a checklist for reviewing articles.

Competencies: 18.1–18.5, 19.1–19.12, 20.1–20.6.

Suggested Resource Material

Again, many of the references from the Annotated Bibliography or Reference section would be useful here, particularly:

Day, R. A. (1979). *How to write and publish a scientific paper.* Day's criteria for reviewing a scientific paper are succinct and memorable: (1) Is it new? (2) Is it true? (3) Is it important? (4) Is it intelligible?
Dirckx, J. A. (1977). *Dx and Rx: A physician's guide to medical writing.*
Huth, E. J. (1982). *How to write and publish papers in the medical sciences.*

405. PREPARING A SYLLABUS AND OTHER STUDENT/ PATIENT MATERIALS (One half-day workshop)

Lecture–discussion in tandem with an education consultant focusing on the audience and format issues involved with writing syllabi, student workbooks, and patient education literature. If there are enough participants, and if their purposes are clearly distinct, the group may be split into two sections, one to address syllabi, another to address patient education literature. The two basic issues confronting writers for either product, however, are: (1) determining what information should be included, and (2) presenting information simply, in language that students or patients can understand.

Format guidelines for preparing syllabi should be presented, along with the educational principles supporting these guidelines. Readability formulas and general tips for writing for lay readers could also be presented, along with some exercises in conceptualizing student and patient audiences.

The last third of the class time is devoted to individual projects. Faculty working on syllabi or education leaflets can use this time to consult with the workshop leaders individually, share products with one another, or begin drafting materials based on the format guidelines.

Competencies: 18.1–18.5, 20.1–20.3.

Suggested Resource Material

See the Reference section for complete citations.

Gall, M. D. (1981). *Handbook for evaluating and selecting curriculum materials.* Very good, very complete, although targeted for the elementary/secondary school publishing market.

McConnell, J. V. (1978, February). Confessions of a textbook writer. A natural storyteller who describes the importance of reaching one's audience through parables, anecdotes, and examples. This may be useful for some educational projects.

Office of Medical Studies. (1978). *A manual for generating course syllabi* (Resource Document #3), C. P. Friedman (Ed.). Very helpful format guide.

Zenger, F., & Zenger K. (1973). *Writing and evaluating curriculum guides.* Some useful (if elaborate) formats that have generic appeal.

406. ADMINISTRATIVE WRITING (One full-day workshop)

In this workshop, three aspects of writing are discussed as they apply to letters of correspondence, memos, curriculum vitae, and summary reports. Brief writing exercises are interspersed with lecture-discussion on the three concepts described below.

The first concept concerns tone or style. Correct tone achieves a relationship between the author and the audience. The appropriate use of tact, diplomacy, assertiveness, opinion, and so forth is demonstrated in "upward" and "downward" forms of communication. Examples of different writing styles (e.g., personal, formal, persuasive) are analyzed and practiced in a learning exercise.

The second concept concerns actual coherence. "Good" and "bad" examples of memos and reports are compared to illustrate both clear and cloudy messages. Communications that illuminate "nest steps" are compared with those that seem to leave no prescriptions for action; information that focuses on the important questions or decisions is contrasted with verbiage that obscures the issues.

The third concept concerns model formats for letters, memos, vitae, and executive summaries. Generic outlines indicating what information writers should include, in what order, will be reviewed along side of actual examples.

A Written Performance Inventory (see References below) may be used as a self-evaluation checklist.

Competencies: 18.1–18.5, 19.1–19.6, 20.1–20.3.

Suggested Resource Material

See the Reference Section for complete citations and the Annotated Bibliography for more description.

Donatelle, E. P. (1984). Administrative communication by written correspondence. In R. B. Taylor & K. A. Munning (Eds.), *Written communication in family medicine.* A 4-hour workshop such as the one described above can be based on this chapter and the readings from Fielden (see below).

Fielden, J. S. (1964). What do you mean I can't write?

Fielden, J. S. (1982). What do you mean you don't like my style?

Tichy, H. S. (1966). *Effective writing for engineers, managers, scientists.* See Chapter 15 for sample letter and short business forms.

407. WRITING RETREAT (Either 2 or 3 days)

A residential retreat for authors working on manuscripts, grants, or other large reports. The retreat agenda combines major blocks of time set aside for writing with individual consultation with an author's editor and possibly a research consultant; exchange of papers and peer-group discussion; minilectures; and reading and relaxation.

Guidelines for program design:

- Six weeks before the retreat, require all prospective participants to submit a rough draft of one or more manuscripts to the writing consultant/retreat leader. Papers should be reviewed and returned with suggested revisions. Faculty should arrive at the retreat with revised manuscripts (and questions) in hand. Only faculty whose research projects are essentially finished should attend.
- After initial introductions at the retreat, intersperse free writing time with group critiques, minilectures, and relaxation exercises.
- Incorporate several minilectures (15–30 minutes) on topics such as (1) why publishing is important to the research process, (2) the structure of the medical article, (3) the writing and revision process, and (4) what clear writing sounds like: nouns, verbs, concrete terms.
- During individual consultations, give faculty feedback on their manuscripts and assign them specific tasks to work on during free writing periods.
- Keep discussion groups very small (3–5 people) and provide guidelines for critiquing other people's work (or model ways to give constructive feedback). Circulate papers before and after faculty revise their work, holding at least two small group critiques.
- Bring resource materials along for faculty to read. Include literature that inspires (Lewis Thomas, William Osler, short excerpts from Mark Twain, John McPhee), examples from the medical literature, handbooks on writing, a dictionary, a thesaurus, and other handouts listed under course #401 tip sheets.
- If possible, bring along a secretary, a word processor, or several portable typewriters. A copier is also handy for getting revised papers out to small-group participants to review.
- Conclude the retreat with definite expectations for completed articles (or progress toward same).

- Six weeks after the retreat, follow up with appointments with each faculty participant. Publish the names of all faculty who finish manuscripts (as well as faculty who submit and eventually publish them) in the department newsletter, or post the names in a memo.

Competencies: 19.1–19.5, 20.1–20.6, 21.1–21.24.

Suggested Resource Material

Many of the references already cited are applicable here. King's Chapter 11 in *Why Not Say It Clearly* (1978) describes a week-long course in medical writing that could be condensed into a retreat.

408. FACULTY PUBLISHING GROUP (One hour-long meeting a month)

If a writing consultant or experienced author is on hand, a local faculty publishing group can serve as a supportive network for authors. The purpose of the group is to exchange information on publishing, share and review colleagues' manuscripts, give feedback on early drafts or outlines, discuss obstacles to writing, find new leads into the literature, etc. Sometimes just the opportunity to express ideas or present research findings to an audience can build incentive to finish an article.

A good time to begin a group is after a retreat, because participants have already developed ties with other faculty authors and experienced the benefits of peer critique. Initially the writing consultant can give direction to the group and demonstrate constructive ways to critique a manuscript. The consultant then serves as a resource to the group, providing technical information and instruction on issues as they come up. Over time, the writing consultant transfers more of the editing and consulting tasks to faculty in the group, giving less direct service as others become more skilled and self-directed.

Competencies: All

Suggested Resource Material

Fielden, J. (1964). *What do you mean I can't write?* Has a one-page assessment sheet on page 147 to use when reading a colleague's paper.
King, L. (1978). *Why not say it clearly: A guide to scientific writing.* Editing exercises appear in the chapter "The Craft of Shortening."

Ruggiero, C. W., Elton, C. F., Mullins, C. J., & Smoot, J. G. (1985). Effective writing: Go tell it on the mountain. Contains a smattering of advice on publishing and specific guidelines for using colleague reviewers. It also advises peers on how to speed-edit and give constructive feedback.

Rationale for the Domain Design

Several factors influenced the design of this model. First, our surveys of department chairs, residency directors, graduates, and exemplary medical faculty gave us some clearcut evidence of need (or lack of it) for writing instruction. For example, we found that residency directors and department chairs in family medicine departments considered writing skills essential, but only for tenure-track faculty. The two goals related to writing that these leaders considered essential for success were: (1) communicate results of research by publishing and making presentations, and (2) communicate effectively in administrative writing, student materials, and patient literature. Neither department chairs nor residency directors thought writing skills were essential for non-tenure-track or preceptor faculty.

Similarly, graduates of Robert Wood Johnson (RWJ) and Federal fellowships who are now in non-tenure-track or preceptor faculty positions did not consider writing skills essential for success. Only RWJ alumni considered writing essential for tenure-track positions in university settings. Exemplary faculty in primary care fields showed a similar pattern in their ratings of writing competencies. Preceptors, faculty members, and "star" preceptors found none of the writing competencies essential for success in their settings. non-tenure-track "star" faculty rated only two competencies essential, and tenure-track "star" faculty said 33 were either highly desirable or essential for success.

In sum, these important groups told us that writing competencies were low on the list of priorities for all but tenure-track faculty. We concluded that it would be a rare department or program that would fund more than a brief workshop in writing for non-tenure-track and preceptor faculty, and a rare non-tenure-track faculty member who would commit the necessary time to improve his or her writing. For this reason, the strategies in Written Communication reflect the needs of tenure-track faculty most. Courses and other activities should be available to all interested faculty, however. Readers will find that written communication courses appear as options in two of four implementation plans.

To further pinpoint faculty members' need for writing skills, we

next reviewed the reactions of our faculty and department committee advisors to the requisite competencies. Their reactions to the writing competencies were rather uniform in a particular sense: They felt
it was impossible to separate any subset of competencies from the
whole and assign them to one faculty group (in either setting) or
exclude them from another. Rather, the competencies seemed to be
an integrated net of process skills. For faculty who write even moderate amounts, virtually all the skills are essential. To illustrate: before
writing even one article, an author needs to know for whom one is
writing (1st skill cluster), how to organize and structure thoughts (2nd
skill cluster), how to format material (3rd skill cluster), and how to
compose sentences (4th skill cluster).

Therefore, no major block of written communication competencies suggested by the literature review was dropped. Rather, the curriculum has adopted all of the competencies. The teaching strategies,
however, emphasize certain competencies more than others. This
emphasis is based on several assumptions about the context of faculty
writing, assumptions we formed through personal observation, and
discussions with editors working in family practice departments. The
assumptions are that:

1. The primary reason why tenure-track faculty write is to publish. Therefore, most of the strategies (e.g., courses #402, #404,
   #407, and #408) are oriented to producing scholarly articles,
   and engage and motivate faculty by helping them to do this.
2. To expand upon this, faculty (particularly medical faculty) are
   not usually interested in learning to write for writing's sake.
   They are very interested in learning in their articles, however,
   and are therefore responsive to Barzun and Graft's argument
   that "the expression is the knowledge. What is not properly
   presented is simply *not present*—and its purely potential exis-
   tence is quite useless" (p. xiii, *The Modern Researcher,* 1977).
   Once faculty realize that their ability to think and to communicate is being examined (rather than some arbitrary
   grasp of grammatical trivia), then they are keen to state their
   arguments well.
3. Although all the requisite competencies are important, if an
   editor is available and faculty are writing to only one major
   audience, then the two most important areas in the curriculum are *organizing the message at hand* and *format considerations.* Again, most of the strategies reflect this. There is, for
   example, no "Cadillac" course on English grammar, usage,

style, etc., although the need may be very apparent. Rather, usage and style can be imparted slowly over time during consultation; to a lesser extent these precepts can be absorbed through subliminal instruction and materials (course #401). Least advantageously, but realistically, authors can learn about their errors in style and usage from journal editors when their manuscripts are returned, heavily marked up, for revision.

Other coordinators of faculty development writing programs (e.g., the Minnesota Writing Project) lend support to this approach. They advise editors to work last on matters of grammar and usage, particularly when this is the adult learner's major area of weakness. Other editors agree; in the first face-to-face consult they suggest returning an author's manuscript clean (with no corrections of any kind) and a very short list of questions written on a separate paper. Only after authors have conceptualized their material and perhaps written several short drafts should the editor closely copyedit the paper.

A final set of factors we considered in designing this domain concerns the overarching delivery system—the best overall way to get knowledge and skills from person or source A to persons B, C, and D.

Ideally, the best way to provide faculty with the guided practice, feedback, and time they need to write is to have a full-time staff writing consultant. A shared appointment with another department may be possible if costs must be kept down. But ongoing, individual consultation—supplemented with intense, working retreats and short, targeted seminars—seems to be the most effective combination of teaching strategies possible. Subliminal instruction tactics and materials may not make much of an impact alone, but they can remind faculty of a consultant's presence and provide a modest antidote to the epidemic of humorless, bad writing that plagues academic communities.

If departments cannot afford a full-time consultant or share one with other departments, it may be possible to get a hospital's public relations staff member to copyedit manuscripts on a freelance basis. This function is a much-reduced version of the consultant's role described in course #402.

Without a staff editor or seasoned author about (and one who is generous with his/her time, to boot), faculty are left to import writing consultants to conduct retreats and seminars as outlined in courses #403, #404, #405, #406, and #407 and to attend national workshops or conferences (see Additional Resources). In the latter strategy, opportunities for personal attention on individual manuscripts are quite

diminished. The most crucial aspect in this instructional task—
ongoing practice, feedback, and support—is lost.

For this reason, we strongly suggest that departments add a writing consultant to the staff of any fellowship or faculty development
program designed to train tenure-track faculty. Perhaps a shared
appointment for an English professor or contract work with an editor from the local university press could help fill the gap if staff
resources are tight. Otherwise, most faculty will be forced to learn
writing "cold turkey" style, a method that may explain why so many
academicians do not write.

Additional Resources

Workshops and Conferences.

Society of Teachers of Family Medicine. Writing workshops and seminars have
been offered during their annual spring meetings, predoctoral meetings, and at faculty development workshops sponsored by Robert Taylor,
M.D., and Joseph Scherger, M.D. Sessions have focused on the medical
article, its structure and language. Well recommended. For more information contact Susie Butler at STFM, (800) 274–2237, or Robert Taylor (Professor and Chairman) at the Oregon Health Science's University
School of Medicine, Department of Family Medicine, 3181 Southwest
Sam Jackson Park Road, Portland, OR 97201, (503) 225–7590.
American Medical Writers Association. Annual Conferences with excellent
writing and editing workshops scheduled for novices and experts. Special education programs tailored for groups and organizations. Although
the Association serves professional writers more than academic faculty,
the skills training in their "core curriculum" sequence looks excellent.
Contact: Lillian Sablack, Executive Director, AMWA, 5272 River Road,
Suite 410, Bethesda, MD 20816, (301) 986–9119.

Workshop Materials.

Scherger, J. E., & Taylor, R. B. *Writing a medical article* (seven pages). Contact Dr. Taylor (see above).
Taylor, R. B. *Biomedical writing workshop* (six pages). Contains objectives;
discussion outline; exercise sheets in organization, composition, and editing; and references.
Taylor, R. B. *Biomedical writing: A perspective.* A 13-page overview of writing formats, the writing process, and steps to publication. Additional
materials included annotated references and handouts for: (1) model
research protocol, (2) reference style, (3) permission requests, (4) the nuts
and bolts of copyright, (5) table of proofreader's marks, and (6) workshop handouts.

Annotated Bibliography

The references below were considered especially important to the content expert in defining and developing this domain. Therefore, they have been annotated, while other cited works have been included only in the Reference section. (For complete citations of these annotations and all other writings mentioned in this domain, turn to the Reference section at the end of this chapter.) Annotations can be very illuminating to readers for a number of reasons. First, they give readers who are not particularly familiar with the subject matter some important background information—a kind of "Cliff's Notes" to the curriculum content. Second, many of the annotations point to specific chapters or excerpts that may stimulate "quick-and-dirty" teaching materials. Third, they can help direct whatever further literature searches you may be planning in the area on your own.

Last, but not least, the discerning reader will learn much about the content expert's vision, perspective, or philosophic stance regarding his or her subject by reading these deliberately selected annotations. Perhaps even more than the prose in the section above, this bibliography may help you to see the subject matter as the content expert saw it and to understand why the domain is structured the way it is.

Altick, R. D. (1969). *Preface to critical reading.*

This is a superb textbook on how to read critically and write intelligibly. Its central request is that we subject all texts to the same intense treatment we give a love letter, when (in Mortimer Adler's words) people ". . . read for all they are worth":

> They read every word three ways: they read between the lines and in the margins; they read the whole in terms of the parts, and each part in terms of the whole; they grow sensitive to context and ambiguity, to insinuation and implication. . . . Then, if never before or after, they read. (Adler, 1940, p. 14)

Altick is analytical, precise, and insightful, yet he approaches the task of teaching critical reading with imagination—no dry text analyses here. In this approach reading and writing assignments are combined. In fact, apart from the foreword (which constitutes a rationale for reading), the book appears to be on writing. Chapters cover the domain of rhetoric quite thoroughly: denotation and connotation of words, diction, determinants of tone, sentences and paragraphs. His final chapter, "Patterns of Clear Thinking," is important for researchers and scholars, as it discusses inductive and deductive reasoning, detection of fallacies, invalid inferences, and other groundless assertions.

Throughout the text lie marvelous examples taken from advertising, journalism, poetry, "great thinkers," literary masters, and bureaucrats. A good quarter of the book consists of specific writing exercises, which makes this volume useful to faculty developers in addition to supporting the competencies.

Barzun, J. (1975). *Simple and direct: A rhetoric for writers.*

This is a very readable handbook for writers, complete with short reading excerpts and writing exercises. It also supports many of the competencies related to audience, organizing content, and usage, style, and composition. Barzun's chapter titles reveal much about his approach to content:

- Diction, or Which Words to Use?
- Linking, or What to Put Next?
- Tone and Tune, or What Impression Will It Make?
- Meaning, or What Do I Want to Say?
- Composition, or How Does It Hang Together?
- Revision, or What Have I Actually Said?

Barzun is a well-known author whose work *The Modern Researcher* (co-authored by H. Graff, 1977) is a respected treatise on the importance of literature and writing to research. Nonetheless, his writing exemplifies a style rarely found in the research literature. It is simple, direct, and clearly expressive. His manner of explaining the decisions we face in writing (e.g., Which word? Which sentence construction? Which sequence of ideas?) is nonacademic, free of dogma. Rather it is guided by the sound, the sense, and the meaning of words selected to represent our thoughts.

Boice, R., & Ferdinand, J. (1984). *Why academicians don't write.*

Lest faculty in academic medicine feel alone in their reluctance to write for publication, consider this important and thorough review of research on writing in higher education. This paper examines the factors that discourage writers, critiques the editorial process, and summarizes literature from composition research. It catalogues the reasons why faculty do not write, the attributes of faculty who do, and strategies for initiating and sustaining writing momentum.

Interestingly, most academicians who do write contribute infrequently. "As few as 10 percent of writers in specific areas account for over 50 percent of the literature" (p. 567). "The median number of . . . publications for even the most prolific disciplines like psychology is zero" (p. 567). The most common reasons given for not publishing are lack of time and competing priorities, yet "surveys indicate that academicians who write have no more free time or no fewer commitments . . . than colleagues who do not" (p. 569). Successful writers simply make time; they preoccupy themselves with ideas about writing almost daily.

Writing blocks do account for a certain lack of productivity. Early negative experiences, delusions of grandiosity and perfectionism, writing anxiety, and negative self-talk contribute to blocked performance. Keys to penetrating such blocks are systematic and frequent writing sessions. Rather than resembling stereotypes of feverishly creative authors, successful academic writers are organized, hard-working, and able to produce in limited amounts of time. Additional qualities include: (1) readiness to accept rejection and to resubmit work to less prestigious journals, (2) ability to respond to criticism rationally (especially when it is unfair), and (3) willingness to edit, revise, and learn from evaluations.

The competencies specified for the Written Communication domain reflect many of the findings and attitudes of this paper. Faculty developers and writing consultants will find the 111 citations listed useful.

Corbett, E. P. J. (1977). *The little rhetoric and handbook.*

Corbett's orientation is to students taking freshman composition, but his content spans the domain of English rhetoric, the fundamentals of which support all the areas in Written Communication.

In two primary chapters, "Finding Something to Say" and "Selecting and Organizing the Material," the author presents various paradigms for investigating subject areas and shows how these paradigms influence the outline of the paper. In this way, the journalist's formula or "who, what, when, where, why, and how," for example, guides the generation and development of content as well as the presentation format. Other paradigms and common patterns of compositional order are discussed.

In these and a later chapter, Corbett also provides structure to the writing process. The first draft of any product—letter, report, or syllabus—should be considered prewriting, or "writing for discovery." Revisions for final drafts are subsequent steps in a systematic process of refinement and clarification. Corbett teaches sentence structure and paragraph development by presenting contrasting examples and asking students to imitate them. This chapter may be especially useful to faculty developers or editors working with authors on sentence patterns and composition.

Dirckx, J. H. (1977). *Dx and Rx: A physician's guide to medical writing.*

Dirckx is a physician and writer who possesses considerable knowledge about language and skill in writing. Essentially, the book is about usage, style, and composition as they apply to the scholarly article, but he deals with critical reading, the derivation of words, "voice," and audience concerns as well. A chapter on accuracy deals with frequent flaws in the medical literature, such as hedging (overqualifying), pompous writing, "writing around the truth," not knowing the literature cited, faulty logic (inductive and deductive reasoning), and bias. His "reading diet for physicians" includes Ralph Waldo Emerson, Oliver Wendell Holmes, Sir William Osler, Charles Darwin, and Thomas Huxley. His list of frequently misspelled medical terms would make a handy handout to offer faculty authors.

Fielden, J. (1964). *What do you mean I can't write?*

In this article, writing style and readability are discussed from the business manager's point of view. Like the academic medical administrator, business professionals have to transmit policy, build alliances, negotiate financial contracts, define jobs, and more through the medium of words. Noting that subscribers to *Harvard Business Review* rate "the ability to communicate" as the number one characteristic influencing a manager's promotion, the author says, "it's time to define what good business writing really is."

Whether the format is letter, memo, or report, the four prized virtues of good business writing are readability, correctness, appropriateness, and thought. The author explains each of these categories in the text. They have been assembled into a "Written Performance

Inventory" as well; this is an evaluative checklist (to use with peers, subordinates, or oneself) to identify writing problems.

Essentially, *readability* concerns presenting information on a level that readers can understand, and in a format that makes it easy to grasp. Unnecessarily abstract words, jargon, and specialized terms frustrate readers at an introductory knowledge level. Similarly, lack of transitions, introductions, summaries, and poor composition generally make it difficult for readers to receive the intended message.

Correctness denotes the mechanics of grammar, punctuation, format, and general coherence. Failure to use an established company form or stating information inaccurately fall into this category.

Appropriateness concerns the proper attitudes of the writer as expressed in his/her "tone of voice." Fielden spends more time on this subtle but important concept in "What do you mean you don't like my style?" but the distinction between *upward* and *downward* communication is well explained here.

Thought attends to overall clarity and competence with the subject matter. Whether the author has prepared his/her topic well, carried out an assignment faithfully, analyzed the data correctly, and prepared the message persuasively are assessed in this category.

Much of faculty writing comes under the administrative heading. Practical guidelines and standards do differ from those described for scholarly writing. Fielden's inventory is a good introduction to this area.

Hayes, J. R., & Flower, L. S. (1986). *Writing research and the writer.*

An excellent overview of the "process movement" in writing instruction and the research on cognitive processes of writing. Together with Scardamalia and Bereiter's (1986) chapter, "Research on Written Composition" (see References), this article provides an excellent gateway to a very active research area.

Cognitive theorists began to look closely at the information processing skills required in writing about 15 years ago. Hayes's and Flower's model of the composing process is probably the most widely cited of the several proposed. This model conceives of writing as an interactive event engaging the author's *knowledge* (stored in long-term memory) with the *task environment* (the "stimulus" and constraints of a "problem") through an interactive process of *planning, text generation,* and *revision.*

The important contribution to teaching practices occurs within this latter component. Teachers in the process movement attempt to explain the "internal" events of writing. Activities are designed to help students develop process skills such as (1) generating content (brainstorming), (2) organization (mapping or outlining), (3) goal setting, (4) casting information into sentences, paragraphs, and larger units, (5) gathering early feedback from members of the writer's audience, and (6) revising material in a cyclic rather than linear fashion.

The research findings presented in this article pertain to the three processes of planning, text generation, and revision. Many of the findings come from studies comparing expert and novice writers using "thinking aloud protocols." Some interesting results are that good writing is very goal-directed; although modifying goals may be essential, goals themselves become hierarchically ordered and perform the function of "driving" the generation and revision of content. In terms of revision, "the more expert the writer, the greater the proportion of writing time the writer will spend in revision" (p. 1110).

This body of research is having a profound effect on writing instruction. One recent meta-analysis (Hillocks, 1984) suggests that process-oriented instruction "is already more successful than previous product-oriented instruction." This may be especially true with novice writers.

Huth, E. J. (1982). *How to write and publish papers in the medical sciences.*

Chapter 1 of this book, "The Paper, the Audience, and the Right Journal," immediately targets three areas in our domain and the essential tasks awaiting authors in academic medicine: identifying and speaking to a specific audience, developing and organizing content, and drafting content according to a prescribed format. Different types of articles are presented and defined, including the case report, literature review, editorial, book review, and letters-to-the-editor, as well as the experimental study.

Another noteworthy chapter is "Revising Prose Style." Here all the elements of usage, style, and composition are addressed: spelling, verb tense, piled-up modifiers, misplaced or dangling modifiers, ambiguous antecedents, empty phrases and for words, "sex-referenced" language, pomposity, and slang. Revising for brevity and clarity as well as a general scheme for revising sentences and paragraphs are also covered.

Huth's central message concerning research articles is that you can not get a good paper out of poor research, and poor writing reflects weak critical thinking skills. A section on searching the literature should help faculty during the prewriting stage.

King, L. S. (1978). *Why not say it clearly: A guide to scientific writing.*

A highly regarded, celebrated book by the former senior editor of the Journal of the American Medical Association. King developed this material ("his personal credo") after 16 years of editing and teaching medical writing. His stated goals for this volume are "to induce in the reader the ability to discriminate good writing from bad, to develop a gut reaction against whatever is clumsy and unclear, to identify specific factors that make bad writing bad, and then to effect improvement."

The author begins by sensitizing the reader's ear to awkward phrasing, improper construction, and muddy thinking. He moves next to "Five Treacherous Servants," an excellently compacted lesson in grammar, covering multiple writing flaws as they occur in connection with the words *is, of, and, very,* and *it.*

Finally, King concludes with advice to the teacher or consultant in setting up a course on medical writing. Consultants, editors, and faculty developers will find this section particularly useful. All faculty authors should have a copy of this book. It does an excellent job of analyzing writing style and giving readers a feel for clear, strong prose.

McLaughlin, G. H. (1969). *SMOG grading—A new readability formula.*

To the question "What characteristics of written text make it difficult for people to read?" psycholinguistic researchers answer, "Word and sentence length." This is because, in English, longer words tend to have more precise meanings; "so a reader must make extra effort. . . to identify the full meaning of a long word, simply because it is precise" (p. 640). Similarly, long sentences tend to have more complex grammatical structures, which "strain the reader's immediate memory because he has to retain several parts of each sentence. . . to combine them into a meaningful whole" (p. 642).

A variety of readability formulas exist. The one presented by McLaughlin, the SMOG (not an acronym but a tribute to the author's home town of foggy London) measures the difficulty level of written text by counting the number of polysyllabic words in a sample of 30 sentences. (All words of three syllables or more are counted.) The square root of the total (rounded to the nearest perfect square) yields the readability score. This score equals the grade level necessary in order to understand the text.

Reading formulas in general are somewhat controversial, although educational publishers depend on them heavily to tailor curricula to specific grade levels. Nonetheless, the practice of moderating one's language to suit the audience cannot be encouraged too highly. Faculty who write for patients, students, staff, and even colleagues (who often read professional journals at home, late at night) should apply the formula to their own writing. Readers please note: Bradley and Currie, writing in *Written Communication in Family Medicine* (STFM Task Force on Professional Communication Skills, 1984), caution that "patients will probably need to have finished two to three more years of school" to read at the level indicated by the formula. Writers are also advised to write at the seventh- or eight-grade level whenever writing for the general public.

Society of Teachers of Family Medicine Task Force on Professional Communication Skills (1984). *Written communication in family medicine.*

A text written specifically for faculty in a primary care specialty, this volume is an excellent gateway to the important subdomains and publication types of academic medical writing. An initial survey of STFM members revealed that faculty's greatest needs lay in written (as opposed to oral) communication skills and that their needs were not confined to research articles and books. Basing their work on these results, the authors examine a full range of writing opportunities from patient education to grant writing to administrative communication. It also supplies writers with insights on the writing and editorial processes, guidelines on style rules and composition, and tips on publication sources and supplementary reading. The broad focus and introductory nature of the work can be seen by scanning the table of contents: "Elements of composition"; On writing: "Getting started, getting stuck, and getting finished"; "Writing a medical article"; "Seeking publication"; "Writing for communication with the public"; "Administrative communication"; "Grant getting"; "Curriculum and instructional applications"; "Writing patient education materials"; "The editorial process in *Family Medicine*"; "Selected publishing sources in family medicine"; a short, annotated bibliography for authors of medical, scientific, and other scholarly articles.

Strunk, W., Jr., & White, E. B. (1979). *The elements of style.*

Probably the single most frequently cited style book in publishing today, this classic practices what it preaches: clear, succinct, graceful prose. The book was originally written in 1918 by Strunk, an English professor at Cornell University and White's teacher and mentor, then revised and expanded by White.

White explains that the book does not "pretend to survey the whole field. Rather it proposes to give in brief space the principal requirements of plain English style. It concentrates on fundamentals: the rules of usage and principles of composition most commonly violated" (p. xii). The authors achieve this by listing rules on usage, composition, and form. Each rule is illustrated with "good" and "bad" examples.

Although the book may seem geared more to writers of fiction, essays, or narrative accounts than medical research, it has high practical value. If writers can avoid making the mistakes listed here, they will have mastered between 80% and 90% of their technical writing problems.

Tichy, H. S. (1966). *Effective writing for engineers, managers, scientists.*

A lively text on technical writing that covers in depth topics such as the writing process, composition, grammar, style, editing, and specific letter and report formats.

Tichy has effectively translated her knowledge of English to the applied worlds of science and industry. She speaks to her audience with obvious knowledge of their concerns. Still, the work is probably most valuable for the faculty developer. teacher, or medical editor rather than beginning writers, because it presumes greater knowledge and appreciation for language than most faculty possess. In terms of rendering the domain of writing into a complete didactic model, however, this work is one of the finest. As such, it guided many (if not most) of the stated competencies in this domain.

Some highlights can be found in Chapters 7 ("Fallacies to Forget") and 8 ("Brevity: The Soul of It"). Here Tichy discusses common misconceptions and suggests ways to delete extraneous words, sentences, and paragraphs. Chapter 9 ("The Standard of Grammar for the Professions") explains how words relate to one another and function in a sentence. Her examples of letter and short business forms (Chapter 15) are excellent models of administrative writing; the prototype "letter of condolence" should be read by anyone needing to convey formal sympathy to a colleague or employee.

And finally, Tichy sympathetically treats the difficult process of beginning to write ("Two Dozen Ways to Begin"). In fact, her first six chapters discuss prewriting activities, outlining, and using a format to advantage.

University of Chicago. (1982). *A manual of style.*

This twelfth, revised edition is a classic, building upon the foundation of previous University of Chicago style manuals, the earliest of which was published for the public in 1906. Its three main sections cover bookmaking, style, and production (printing). By style, the editors mean "house rules" for punctuation, spelling, names and terms, numbers, foreign languages, quotations, captions, tables, mathematics, abbreviations, notes and footnotes, bibliographies, citations of public documents, and indexes. It serves authors and editors well as a reference book once they have learned how to access it. In conjunction with *The Elements of Style*, it was the main source for competencies listed under usage, style, and composition.

Woodford, F. P. (1967). *Sounder thinking through clearer writing.*

Several authors address the relationship between critical thinking, reading, and writing skills, but no one states the case more forcibly than Woodford does here. In this author's view:

> Bad scientific writing involves more than stylistic inelegance: it is often the outward and visible form of an inward confusion of thought. The scientific literature at its present standard distorts rather than forms the graduate student's view of scientific knowledge and thought, and corrupts his ability to write, to read, and to think (p. 745).

Woodford begins by listing that which is bad in scientific writing: vague nouns, "scientific impartiality" (use of the passive voice), polysyllabic terms, ungrammatical constructions, jargon, pompous language, concealed hedging, unjustifiable interpretations, ambiguity, and confused thought.

Although he illustrates his point with humorous examples (e.g., students "no longer walk through a door without 'utilizing a pedestrian relocation'"). Woodford's argument is serious. Having observed the quality of students' thinking deteriorate with their exposure to poor scientific writing, he uses writing as a tool to sharpen their critical thinking and reading skills. Woodford asserts that "[T]he power of writing as an aid in thinking is not often appreciated. . . . the very act of writing can help to clarify thinking (p. 744).

Woodford believes the purpose of a graduate course on scientific writing should be to strengthen scientific thinking; he teaches such a course, contending it belongs "at the very heart of a scientific curriculum." Suggested course topics include: (1) separating main issues from side issues and irrelevancies, (2) the function of publication, (3) methods of literature search, (4) the nature of scientific proof, and (5) a sense of style.

The faculty developer or writing consultant will find support for his/her efforts here.

Ziman, J. M. (1969). *Information, communication, knowledge.*

The nature of scientific communication is held up for review and commentary in this article. According to Ziman, the aim of science is to "create, criticize, or contribute to a rational consensus of ideas and information." As such, the research paper is the point at which those ideas are tested and absorbed into the public scientific domain.

The author goes on to describe three basic characteristics of the "primary" literature. First, the literature is fragmentary, consisting of many discrete pieces of scientific work carried out by individuals cooperating in a larger corporate enterprise. This means that "a typical scientific paper has never pretended to be more than another little piece in a larger jigsaw—not significant in itself but as an element in a grander scheme" (p. 318).

Second, scientific literature is derivative because articles are naturally embedded in a context of previous achievements and current activity: "Indeed, one relies on the citations to show its place in the whole scientific structure, just as one relies on a man's kinship affiliations to show his place in his tribe" (p. 318).

Third, the literature is highly "edited," both in terms of censorship (by editorial and peer review) and the writing process itself. By this Ziman means that the "real experience" of conducting research is highly formalized into a research article package that "is not a candid autobiography but a cunningly contrived piece of rhetoric." Hiding all the false starts, unnecessary complications, and mistakes, writers work to spin "a yarn of preternatural prescience, precision, and profit. [The journal article] has only one purpose; it must persuade the reader of the veracity of the observer, his disinterestedness, his logical infallibility, and the complete necessity of his conclusions" (p. 319). Although this interpretation casts a satirical eye on research and publishing, it remains essentially correct. Good writing is goal-driven, deliberate distillation and ordering of experience.

In the remainder of the paper, Ziman discusses the necessity of referees (peer review), delays in communicating scientific research, possibilities for informal information exchanges and networks, and future technologies for indexing and disseminating printed material. Along the way he provides a very nice definition of a good review article and the contribution it can make to "sifting and sorting out" primary observations in the larger pattern.

"Literature" as a concept is an important one for beginning researchers and writers to grasp. Often faculty will see data analysis as the end point of research and literature as the subsidiary product of faculty (less busy than themselves!) who have the time to "write up their results." Ziman's article should open this subject up for discussion.

References

Adler, M. (1940). *How to read a book.* New York: Simon & Schuster.

Altick, R. D. (1969). *Preface to critical reading* (5th ed.). New York: Holt, Rinehart, & Winston.

Baker, S. (1984). *The complete stylist and handbook.* New York: Harper & Row.

Barzun, J. (1975). *Simple and direct: A rhetoric for writers.* New York: Harper & Row.

Barzun, J. & Graft, H. (1957). *The modern researcher* (3rd ed.). New York: Harcourt Brace Jovanovich.

Bland, C. J. (1987). *Grant-getting: A workshop for the Society of Teachers of Family Medicine* (personal teaching materials). Minneapolis: University of Minnesota.

Bland, C. J., & Moo-Dodge, M. (1984). Grant-getting. In R. B. Taylor & K. A. Munning (Eds.), *Written communication in family medicine.* New York: Springer-Verlag.

Boice, R., & Ferdinand, J. (1984). Why academicians don't write. *Journal of Higher Education, 55*(5), 567–582.

Corbett, E. P. J. (1977). *The little rhetoric and handbook.* New York: John Wiley & Sons.

Day, R. A. (1979). *How to write and publish a scientific paper.* Philadelphia: ISI Press.

DeBakey, L. (1977, July/August). The persuasive proposal. *Foundation News,* 19–27.

Dirckx, J. H. (1977). *Dx and Rx: A physician's guide to medical writing.* Boston: G. H. Hall.

Donatelle, E. P. (1984). Administrative communication by written correspondence. In R. B. Taylor & K. A. Munning (Eds.), *Written communication in family medicine.* New York: Springer-Verlag.

Fielden, J. (1964, May–June). What do you mean I can't write? *Harvard Business Review,* 144–152.

Fielden, J. (1982, May–June). What do you mean you don't like my style? *Harvard Business Review,* 128–138.

Flower, L. S., & Hayes, J. R. (1981). A cognitive process theory of writing. *College Composition and Communication, 32,* 365–387.

Friedman, C. P. (1978). A manual for generating course syllabi. Resource Document #3, in-house publication. Chapel Hill: University of North Carolina, Office of Medical Studies.

Gall, M. D. (1981). *Handbook for evaluating and selecting curriculum materials.* Boston: Allyn & Bacon.

Gordon, K. E. (1983). *The well-tempered sentence: A punctuation handbook for the innocent, the eager, and the doomed.* New Haven and New York: Tichnor & Fields.

Gordon, K. E. (1984). *The transitive vampire: A handbook of grammar for the innocent, the eager, and the doomed.* New York: Times Books.

Graves, R., & Hodge, A. (1979). *The reader over your shoulder: A handbook for writers of English prose* (2nd ed.). New York: Vintage Books.

Gray, J., & Meyers, M. (1978). The Bay Area Writing Project. *Phi Delta Kappan, 59,* 410–413.

Hayes, J. R., & Flower, L. S. (1986). Writing research and the writer. *American Psychologist, 41*(10), 1106–1113.

Hennessey, J. L. (1977, July/August). The unpersuasive proposal. *Foundation News,* 28–30.

Hillocks, G. (1984). What works in teaching composition: A meta-analysis of experimental treatment studies. *American Journal of Education, 93,* 133–170.

Huth, E. J. (1982). *How to write and publish papers in the medical sciences.* Philadelphia: ISI Press.

International Committee of Medical Journal Editors. (1982). Uniform requirements for manuscripts submitted to biomedical journals. *Annals of Internal Medicine, 96*(Part I), 766–772.

King, L. S. (1978). *Why not say it clearly: A guide to scientific writing.* Boston: Little, Brown.

Kurzig, C. M. (1980). *Foundation fundamentals: A guide for grant seekers.* New York: Foundation Center.

McConnell, J. V. (1978, February). Confessions of a textbook writer. *American Psychologist, 33*(2), 159–169.

McLaughlin, G. H. (1969). SMOG grading—A new readability formula. *Journal of Reading, 969*(2), 639–646.

Reif-Leher, L. (1982). *Writing a successful grant application.* Boston: Science Books International.

Rico, G., & Claggett, M. F. (1980). *Balancing the hemispheres: Brain research and the teaching of writing* (Curriculum Publication 14). Berkeley: University of California Bay Area Writing Project.

Ruggiero, C. W., Elton, C. F., Mullins, C. J., & Smoot, J. G. (1985). Effective writing: Go tell it on the mountain. *The AIR Professional File* (Association for Institutional Research), *21*, 1–7.

Scardamalia, M., & Bereiter, C. (1986). Research on written composition. In M. S. Wittrock (Ed.), *Handbook of research on teaching* (3rd ed.). New York: Macmillan.

Scherger, J. E., & Taylor, R. N. (1984). Writing a medical article. Workshop materials of Robert Taylor, Professor and Chairman, Oregon Health Sciences, University School of Medicine, Department of Family Medicine, 3181 Southwest Sam Jackson Park Road, Portland, OR 97201.

Society of Teachers of Family Medicine Task Force on Professional Communication Skills. (1984). In R. B. Taylor & K. A. Munning (Eds.), *Written communication in family medicine.* New York: Springer-Verlag.

Strunk, W., Jr., & White, E. G. (1979). *The elements of style* (3rd ed.). New York: Macmillan.

Tichy, H. S. (1966). *Effective writing for engineers, managers, scientists.* New York: John Wiley & Sons.

University of Chicago Press. (1982). *A manual of style* (13th ed.). Chicago: University of Chicago Press.

Waddell, M. L., Esch, R. M., & Walker, R. R. (1972). *The art of styling sentences: Twenty patterns to success.* Woodbury, NY: Barron's Educational Series.

Webster's New Collegiate Dictionary. (1973). Springfield, MA: G. & C. Merriam Company.

White, V. P. (1975). *Grants: How to find out about them and what to do next.* New York: Plenum Press.

Woodford, F. P. (1967). Sounder thinking through clearer writing. *Science, 156,* 743–745.

Woodford, F. P. (1968). *Scientific writing for graduate students: A manual on the teaching of scientific writing.* New York: The Rockefeller University Press.

Young, A. (1979, March). *Teaching writing across the university: The Michigan Tech experience.* Paper presented at the Annual Meeting of the College English Association, Savannah, GA.

Zenger, F., & Zenger, K. (1973). *Writing and evaluating curriculum guides.* Belmont, CA: Siegler, McFearson.

Ziman, J. M. (1969). Information, communication, knowledge. *Nature, 224,* 318–324.

CHAPTER **7**

Professional Academic Skills Domain

Introduction to the Domain

The usual advice given to new faculty members trying to adjust to life in academic medicine is to maintain their clinical skills and to develop skills in teaching and research. Occasionally administrative skills (e.g., time management, project administration) are added. This is good advice, but it is insufficient. It is now clear that the successful academician, particularly the researcher, has also acquired certain values, networks and behaviors that are not addressed in the usual faculty development curriculum. In addition, the successful academician also has a supportive work environment. These additional personal and environmental qualities are what distinguish the productive professional academic from the less productive (Bland & Schmitz, 1986). This curriculum does not explain how to establish a supportive work environment. As mentioned before, however, it is such a critical (if not essential) factor in achieving faculty development and continued productivity that we discuss it under philosophy. This section does address how to acquire the additional personal characteristics—what we call professional academic skills—of the successful academician.

Definition of the Professional Academic Skills Domain

All professions are characterized by a unique set of unwritten norms, rules, and practices. Effective attorneys, scientists, priests, and physicians know more than law, science, religion, or medicine. They have learned many unwritten rules, concepts, and behaviors that allow them

to "act like an attorney" or "think like a scientist." They have acquired
the professional attitudes and social skills of their chosen occupation.
These skills include a ". . . somewhat special language, an ideology
that helps edit a member's everyday experience, shared standards of
relevance as to the critical aspects of the work that is being accomplished, matter-of-fact prejudices, models for social etiquette and
demeanor, certain customs and rituals suggestive of how members are
to relate to colleagues, subordinates, superiors, and outsiders. . ." (Van
Maanen & Schein, 1979, p. 210).

These skills are not usually learned through formal instruction
but through a process called *socialization.* "Socialization is a mechanism through which new members learn the values, norms, knowledge,
beliefs, and the interpersonal and other skills that facilitate role performance and further group goals" (Mortimer & Simmons, 1978, p. 423).
In addition to facilitating effective performance, socialization is the
means for ". . . developing commitment to work, for stimulating motivation, and for internalizing occupationally relevant attitudes and
behavior that sustain productivity and continued achievement throughout the career" (Clark & Corcoran, 1986, p. 23). This second outcome
of socialization is especially important for professional academics and
the organizations that employ them. Faculty typically stay in their
profession for a lifetime, and institutions provide them tenure on the
premise that they will remain productive over that lifetime.

A great deal has been written about the importance of socialization. Early writings focused primarily on the cultural socialization that
occurs in childhood. After 1970, the literature shifted to socialization
processes occurring in adulthood (e.g., Hill & Aldous, 1969; Moore, 1969;
Neugarten, 1968). Researchers in this area have been particularly
interested in socialization to professions and organizations (e.g., Bucher
& Stelling, 1977; Dubin, 1976; Mortimer & Simmons, 1978; Nyre &
Reilly, 1979; Van Maanen & Schein, 1979). Competencies slated for this
domain are based primarily on the research findings of Corcoran and
Clark (1984), Pelz and Andrews (1966), Creswell (1985), Bland and
Schmitz (1986), Aran and Ben-David (1968), and others studying the
career development of exceptionally productive faculty as well as those
who were less successful.

Rationale for Including Professional Academic Skills in the Curriculum

Virtually all these studies conclude that socialization is critical for effective performance in a profession and in an organization. Conway and
Glass (1978), in "Socialization for Survival in the Academic World," state:

"If the faculty of a given school wish to see that school ranked among the acknowledged best in the university, the socialization of each new faculty member must become a concern of the corporate body." This finding alone suggest that socialization is an area to which faculty development programs should attend. In specific terms, Creswell (1986), in his extensive review of 130 studies on faculty research productivity, found socialization to be a fundamental career event in predicting scientific productivity. In study after study, socialization factors were both the critical feature and the eventual characteristic that differentiated highly productive from less productive faculty. In most of these studies, productivity was measured by publications. Even in studies where "highly productive" is defined more broadly, however, socialization appears to predict which faculty members will be achievers and those who will not.

In Corcoran and Clark's (1984) work, for example, "highly active" was measured by (1) reputation among colleagues and administrators for excellent teaching and research, and (2) contributions to university governance. Random sampling procedures produced a representative group of faculty matched in age, rank, and discipline to the "highly active" group. The investigators found striking differences in the socialization patterns of the "highly active" and "representative" groups. Highly active faculty said research attracted them to academe, while representative faculty said teaching was most appealing. Highly active faculty said academic freedom and research were the most satisfying aspects of academe; representative faculty said working with students was most satisfying. Highly active faculty reported learning "how to behave" from their advisors and had many more applied-research-related learning experiences (such as assistantships) during graduate school. They also had established significant professional connections with their advisors/mentors and training peers. After graduation, advisors/mentors helped highly active faculty write grants, offered them positions, and collaborated on papers. Similar instances of continuing help and collaboration acquired during training came from peers. The representative group reported fewer instances of such help from advisors, and their relationships with training peers usually assumed a social rather than professional nature.

Several authors specifically address the importance of socialization when preparing physician investigators. Aran and Ben-David (1968), in "Socialization and Career Patterns as Determinants of Productivity of Medical Researchers," found that ". . . in order to become a researcher a medical doctor must be reoriented or 're-socialized' in a framework different from the one in which he had been trained as a doctor and medical specialist" (p. 210). Similarly, Blackburn and Fox

(1976) found that successful physician faculty in a large research-oriented university had acquired the values of researchers and identified with two professions: academics and private practice.

This general correlation between socialization and productivity was echoed in a recent study of family physician faculty who graduated from fellowship programs (Bland, Hitchcock, Anderson, & Stritter, 1986, 1987). This study found that the characteristics that discriminated productive fellowship alumni from their less productive peers also characterized productive researchers in other fields. In particular, the high value placed on research was a characteristic that predicted levels of productivity.

One additional fact makes socialization an important process to address in a faculty development program for physician faculty. Typically, professionals allot a significant amount of time to initiating new members. Although mentors (or other representatives) do not always overtly articulate rules of conduct and thought for the novice, most professions consciously socialize newcomers through a period of apprenticeship. Clinical rotations and residency programs socialize young practicing physicians. Attorneys spend years as junior or associate members of their firm. Psychologists go through internships and supervised counseling. Academics in higher education spend an average of 7 years in doctoral training, during which time the dissertation experience and tutelage under their advisor socialize them to the values of the university professoriate and the expected activities for faculty.

Some physician faculty members gain academic apprenticeship through fellowships, such as those sponsored by the National Institutes of Health, the Robert Wood Johnson Foundation, or Kaiser Foundation. Also, most physician faculty members enter departments with experienced researchers as senior faculty, who informally socialize junior members. But many primary care faculty members have had no explicit mechanism through which to learn the university system. In 1981, David identified some 100 family medicine fellowships available ranging in duration from 6 weeks to 2 years, but half of these positions were unfilled. Moreover, most were too brief to achieve socialization. Finally, primary care divisions or departments are generally too new to have senior research mentors.

We include professional academic skills in this curriculum, therefore, because (1) they are critical for research productivity, and (2) primary care faculty usually have no vehicle or system for acquiring socialization unless it is formally organized by faculty development.

How the Domain Has Been Structured

To identify the specific professional skills faculty need, we return to the definition of socialization. "Socialization is a mechanism through which new members learn the values, norms, knowledge, beliefs, and the interpersonal and other skills that facilitate role performance and further group goals" (Mortimer & Simmons, 1978, p. 422). For simplicity, we have collapsed this definition into three groups of competencies: (1) academic values, (2) knowledge for managing an academic career, and (3) academic relationships (see Table 7.1).

Academic Values.
Understanding the values, norms, and traditions of the profession and organization in which one works is critical, for it is these elements, rather than shared technical knowledge alone, that bond a group to a profession and allow them to work together effectively. Given a common understanding and view of the world, professionals can overcome knowledge differences and agree on goals and means to an end.

According to Blackburn and Fox's (1976) study of medical faculty, Caffrey's (1969) study of liberal arts schools, and other writers in this area (Rice, 1983), the highly ranked norms of academicians are academic freedom and the priority of research. While these values rank higher for Ph.D.'s than M.D.'s, they are consistently high for academic M.D.'s (Blackburn & Fox, 1976). This difference in rank order may be due to the early emphasis on research in doctoral training, while M.D.'s acquire these values later, on the job and from peers.

TABLE 7.1 Subareas in the Professional Academic Skills Domain

---

Academic Values
- Understanding academic values, norms, traditions
- Resolving value conflicts

Academic Relationships
- Applying knowledge and skills at multiple professional levels
- Building and maintaining relationships

Managing An Academic Career
- Setting personal goals and priorities
- Understanding reward and promotion systems
- Understanding goals and operations of academic workplace
- Identifying own and others' roles and daily activities
- Understanding goals and operations of related external organizations

---

Knowledge for Managing an Academic Career.
Knowledge about one's organization, its structure, governance, rewards, career paths, key players, and so forth, is also essential to participate successfully (Bogdewic, 1986; Dill, 1986a). For the academician this means knowing about the institution's mission, administrative structure, and promotion procedure. Because researchers are affected by factors outside their local institution, their success is also determined by their knowledge of funding organizations, professional organizations, and academic and educational organizations.

Academic Relationships.
Relationship skills that are critical to the successful academician include those with mentors, training peers, and research colleagues (Corcoran & Clark, 1984). For example, individuals who associate early with distinguished scientists or collaborate with them on research projects are more likely themselves to become productive researchers (Cameron & Blackburn, 1981). Blackburn (1979) writes: "Mentorship/sponsorship in the first years is critical for launching a productive career—learning the informal network that supports productivity—the inner workings of professional associations and who the productive people are, for example—is critical, especially in the faculty member's first years" (p. 25–26).

   Aran and Ben-David (1968) found that the medical researchers in their study attached "great importance to their continued contact with the scientists whom they had met during their resocialization. . . [and] that change in productivity following resocialization is indeed a function of the intensity of communication of the researcher with other scientists, i.e., of his induction into the scientific community" (p. 12). Pelz and Andrews (1966), in their classic work on scientists in organizations, found that highly productive scholars maintain frequent contact with colleagues and spend significant time communicating with them via personal correspondence, telephone conversations, visits, and exchange of reprints and unpublished papers.

Assumptions Made in Constructing the Domain

Every professional academic setting and group has its own set of values and unwritten rules that successful members learn. The competencies in this domain, however, focus mainly on the professional academic skills needed by newly recruited faculty in research-oriented settings, where success is measured mainly by research productivity. The reasons for this are: (1) the available literature on faculty socialization addresses only research-oriented faculty, and (2) the greatest role conflicts, caused by the difference between practitioner and academic behaviors and values, occur in research-oriented settings.

As to the available literature, there is both a classic and contemporary collection of writings on the socialization and culture of the successful researcher (e.g., Cresswell, 1985; Dill, 1986a; Hagstrom, 1965; Pelz & Andrews, 1966; Shils, 1983; Sindermann, 1985). These studies consistently identify a unique set of attitudes and abilities found in the productive researcher. Conversely, faculty who are less satisfied and less successful in research institutions do not typically possess these attitudes and abilities. It is, by the way, these studies that also point out the importance of the environment in predicting productivity (e.g., Bland et al., 1986; Corcoran & Clark, 1984). Environment includes such things as the reward structure, management style of the leader, and the productivity and mutual reinforcement of peers. In fact, the environment is probably a more powerful predictor of research productivity than individual researcher characteristics.

As stated earlier, however, developing the organizational leaders and the environment necessary for maintaining research productivity is beyond the scope of this curriculum (although developing individual researchers will eventually influence the entire organization and environment). The importance of the environment is mentioned again here to remind the reader that while developing individuals' skills and attitudes is essential, this alone is insufficient if the goal is to produce and maintain productive researchers.

Individual development remains the focus of this curriculum. Accordingly, this section lists the values, personal management, and relationship abilities needed by individual faculty members. Readers will find this list quite specific—more so than in other domains. Simply put, professional academic competencies needed more detail and more examples than those in other domains, whose terms and meanings are relatively commonplace.

As mentioned above, the skills we have enumerated appear necessary for work in settings where success is measured by research productivity. Thus they are certainly requisite for faculty in research-oriented universities. Unfortunately, while there are studies on faculty in community and liberal arts colleges, there are no studies on the values and professional academic skills needed by faculty in more service- or teaching-oriented medical schools or residency training programs. For faculty in these settings, the reader will need to modify some of the competencies listed. Keep in mind, however, that whatever the organization's values and unwritten rules are, they are critical to know because of their influence on individuals' satisfaction and productivity.

Goals and Competencies

Listed below are the goals and competencies for the Professional Academic Skills domain. This list represents the spectrum of professional academic knowledge and skills required of academicians; it is not broken down by institution or faculty type. For suggestions on how to identify relevant subsets of competencies for preceptors, non-tenure-track, and tenure-track faculty, see Chapter 2.

These goals and competencies were prepared by the content expert after engaging in an extensive literature review, meeting with physician liaisons and advisory committee members, reviewing the results of our three surveys, and discussing the domain with the other authors. The competencies are presented according to each subarea of the domain, as identified in Table 7.1.

Academic Values

GOAL 22.0: Understand the underlying values, traditions, and unwritten behavior codes of academia.

The importance of professional values is not to be underestimated. In addition to providing a basis for efficient work, they communicate basic philosophical beliefs held by people in the profession. (Academics, for example, hold common beliefs about preferred methods of establishing the truth or explaining phenomena.) Knowing the underlying values allows a faculty member to understand why persons in the profession behave as they do; to predict a professional's behavior; and to know how to behave in accordance with others in that profession. Thus understanding academic values allows faculty to apply their skills and direct their activities more effectively. Such understanding also enables faculty to defuse value conflicts.

Faculty should be able to:

22.1. Describe what attracts successful academics to the profession (e.g., opportunities to teach, produce new knowledge, determine own area of investigation, enjoy prestige associated with being a university professor, contribute to society by ensuring an educated populace)

22.2. Discuss values of academicians (e.g., academic freedom, importance of knowledge production, publishing, patient care, student growth and development)

22.3. Describe how these values do or do not permeate policy and mission of the institution (e.g., Regent's Mission Statement, promotion and tenure code, grievance process, dean's priorities for the school, and priority of university)

22.4. Identify unwritten rules and practices of academics (e.g., authorship on articles, establishing collaborative research relationships, soliciting information from potential funding sources)

22.5. Discuss values of practicing physicians (e.g., patient care, family, community health)

22.6. Ascertain how well one's own values match with academic and institutional values

22.7. Identify (and adapt to, when appropriate) different value systems within the department, university, practicing community, National Institutes of Health, etc.

Knowledge for Managing an Academic Career

GOAL 23.0: To effectively manage a productive career in academia.

In most organizations, promotion mechanisms controlled by others advance personnel either automatically (e.g., according to seniority) or selectively (e.g., through invitation to join a medical group). In academic settings, however, individual faculty members are personally responsible for understanding how to advance in the organization. Faculty are expected to understand all levels of their organization and how to play a role in it; be aware of the time frame and criteria for advancement; identify and satisfy advancement criteria; manage their work flow to accommodate professional advancement tasks; maintain a dossier documenting how they meet the criteria; and propose themselves for review and promotion at appropriate times. Occasionally there is help along the way with these various steps. For example, a department head may establish a yearly "contract" with faculty members to guide time management, or a department may provide assistance in preparing a promotion packet. If a faculty member does not advance, however, it is seldom considered the organization's problem; rather, the faculty member is considered at fault. Career management, therefore, is clearly the faculty member's responsibility. In order to manage an academic career, faculty members need to understand how the immediate and related organizations impact their career. At the same time, faculty need to assess their own goals and what is expected of them by others.

Faculty should be able to:

23.1.   Describe the purposes of one's own superordinate struc-
        tures (e.g., college, hospital, university)

23.2.   Explain the role of one's own unit within the larger
        organization's goals and purposes

23.3.   Describe the administrative structure of the unit and
        entire organization, naming key people in it (e.g., depart-
        ment head, dean, vice president, president, board of
        regents, affirmative action officer)

23.4.   Describe faculty authority, governance, and participation
        within the administrative structure, naming key people
        in it (e.g., medical school faculty senate chair, medical
        school senate committees, university senate representa-
        tives from medical school, senate president, senate com-
        mittees, hospital committees)

23.5.   Describe one's roles, assignments, and responsibilities in
        the department, college, hospital, or university

23.6.   Describe other faculty members' and support staff roles
        in these settings

23.7.   Describe daily activities of successful academics (e.g., plan
        and teach courses; read broadly in areas affecting dis-
        cipline and institutions; conduct research; participate in
        local, institution-wide, and national committees and
        review panels; work in multiple sites—office, clinic, hospi-
        tal, on the road)

23.8.   Identify how faculty activities are influenced by the
        explicit and implicit expectations of each level of the
        organization (levels might include unit, department, col-
        lege, hospital, and university. Expectations might include
        "publish 3 articles a year in refereed journals," "acquire
        funding for 50% of salary within 2 years through research
        grants or patient-generated dollars," "teach at all levels
        of medical education," "participate in university gover-
        nance through such things as a senate membership or
        promotion review")

23.9.   Describe rewards of being productive in the organization
        (for academics, this is typically the experience of seeing
        one's work used, local recognition, public recognition,
        contribution to knowledge development, contribution to
        student development, contribution to patient care, oppor-
        tunities to participate to higher level of governance and
        administration, promotion, tenure, salary increase)

23.10. Identify personal goals, interests, and rewards

23.11. Assess how well the organization's goals and expectations match with one's desired activities, goals, and interests

23.12. Identify the required or rewarded products (e.g., publication, grants, awards, promotion packet, patient-generated dollars)

23.13. Identify the maximum time allowed (if one exists) for acquiring rewards (e.g., must be promoted in 7 years or terminated, must acquire grant support in 3 years or salary reduced)

23.14. Identify which levels of the organization control the rewards one values (for example, the department head may expect and reward time devoted to patient care, the university may expect and reward, through promotion and tenure, published articles in refereed journals)

23.15. Identify skills, contacts, and experience one needs to produce valued products

23.16. Develop a promotion packet

23.17. Negotiate assignments, leaves, and responsibilities

23.18. Describe the mission and structure and name the people of major funding sources, professional organizations, and academic organizations

23.19. Describe purpose and publishing policies of relevant publications (both practice-oriented and scholarly)

Academic Relationships

GOAL: 24.0 Establish and maintain in a network of professional colleagues in academia.

The nature of work in an academic culture has paradoxically, both an independent and dependent aspect. For instance, a researcher conducts his or her daily routine quite autonomously, either alone or with a small team. At the same time, however, the researcher is very dependent on the previous work of others to build on and advance the body of knowledge. Also, clinicians apply new knowledge gained in research, as well as offer researchers "laboratories" in which to work. Whether reporting results of research, teaching, or new management techniques, all authors are dependent on others to critique and replicate their work and to maintain the quality of work in the field through grant reviews, refereed journals, conference presentations, and critiques. Because of this interdependence, successful academics have a network of professional colleagues who are vital to their effective performance. These colleagues are usually peers, superiors, or former mentors; they may be located at the same or other institutions. They do such things as provide quick access to the most recent work in the area, serve as "thinking partners" when the researcher is stumped, and open doors to peer review panels.

Faculty should be able to:

24.1. Maintain productive (vs. social) professional relationships with an advisor or mentor(s) and with training peers
24.2. Maintain frequent, substantive contact with productive researchers in one's researach area, both within one's institution and elsewhere
24.3. Seek opportunities to collaborate (e.g., combine resources, personnel, activities, goals) across one's network
24.4. Participate in professional groups and activities associated with the college, hospital, university, discipline, research area, or funding sources

Courses, Strategies, and Resources

Listed below are suggested courses, strategies, and resources for teaching the competencies and achieving the goals in the Professional Academic Skills domain. (Competencies to be achieved by each course or other activity are listed by number after each description.) These activities and sources cover the full range of skills identified in Professional Academic Skills; they are not keyed to specific faculty types at particular institutions. For guidelines on how to select and combine courses in this and other domain(s) for preceptors, non-tenure-track, and tenure-track faculty in different institutions, see Chapter 8.1.

501. PROFESSIONAL DEVELOPMENT (Time varies with type of faculty participants)

This is an ongoing seminar in which faculty discuss how all the other faculty development activities fit into the lifetime role, value system, and career development of a professional academic. For tenure-track faculty in a research-oriented university, this seminar should meet for 2 hours twice a month for the entire training period. For non-tenure-track faculty in research settings, and for tenure-track faculty with less role emphasis on research, the seminar should meet less often, for a total of about 40 hours spread over the training period. Non-tenure-track faculty in community-based settings require even less. A modified, shortened version of the seminar, totaling 16 hours or less, should be spread over the training period. In modifying the seminars, developers will be deleting some of the competencies, and emphasizing some topics more than others, as well as shortening the overall length. The purpose of the seminar series is to help participants to acquire the values of an academician, learn how to guide an academic career productively, and establish the basis of a career-long, professional network.

During each seminar a prepared topic is scheduled, with related learning activities. These topics provide participants with an opportunity to use each other, as colleagues, to test and expand their thinking, and to give and receive mutual support. In addition, spontaneous discussion about participants' faculty development activities, research efforts, future as academicians, or questions about current academic events (e.g., search committees, grievances, promotions) should occur. Toward the latter part of the fellowship, sessions should focus more on participants' own research activities and less on formal topics.

Topics

- What is the mission of the participant's university, health sciences complex, medical school, and primary care department(s)?
- How are these and other entities in the university (e.g., office of research administration, office of equal opportunity and affirmative action, civil service) structured and funded to accomplish these missions?
- Who are the administrative leaders of these entities (vice presidents, deans, program directors, department heads, clinical chiefs, etc.)?
- How do faculty and students participate in governance? Who are the faculty leaders (e.g., senate president, judicial committee chair, executive faculty chair)?
- How is the participant's university (e.g., land grant, urban, private) different from others in terms of mission, rewards, values, faculty roles?
- What are the missions and structures of major funding sources, professional organizations, and academic organizations relevant to primary care researchers?
- What purposes do various publications serve? (i.e., publications that are relevant to academia in general and

those more specifically relevant to faculty members' research areas)
- How are the beliefs, practices, and rewards of the dominant professions (e.g., medicine, law, academics) similar or different?
- What are professional networks and how do they work?

In addition to weekly group discussion, seven learning activities are suggested when addressing these topics.

1. *Presentations by university leaders (administration, research, teaching).* When possible, these presentations and interactions should be held in the office of the guest presenter to acquaint faculty with the entire university. These sessions would be used to inform participants of the presenters' roles in the university and to share their understandings and beliefs about academe and academic professionals.

2. *Assigned reading.* When appropriate, participants should have assigned readings, including selections from publications on general academia (e.g., *The Chronicle of Higher Education* and *Academe—The Bulletin of the AAUP*); the mission statements and constitution of the university and its colleges; the university promotion and tenure code; and selected articles from university publications such as the university and the alumni paper.

3. *Assigned practicums.* Where possible, participants should sit in as observers during important meetings or events (e.g., sessions with regents, major search committee meetings, university senate meetings, senate judicial committee meetings, dean's council of advisors, site visits by NIH, promotion committee meetings). Each participant may not be able to take part in every practicum. Therefore, each participant should report these experiences to the group at the biweekly course session.

4. *Debates.* Participants should debate topics related to the major issues, beliefs, and practices of academe (e.g., directed research vs. self-initiated research; value of research vs. teaching vs. patient care; consulting on "university time"; tenure vs. contract appointments).

5. *Simulations.* Participants should experience important academic practices in simulations (e.g., peer review and critique of articles; promotion packet preparation and review; grievance hearings; grant preparation and review; site visit and peer panel).

6. *Contacts.* Participants should be expected to identify individuals or types of individuals whom they would like to contact for their professional network. Each faculty presenter in the course should also describe their professional network, and explain how it evolved and how it is maintained and used.

7. *Professional meetings.* Participants should attend (and ideally present their work in) two professional academic meetings a year [e.g., The Society of Teachers of Family Medicine (STFM), Society of General Internal Medicine (SGIM), Ambulatory Pediatric Association (APA), North American Primary Care Research Group (NAPCRG), Association of American Medical Colleges (AAMC)]. These trips should be planned as optimal professional experiences as opposed to social outings. A minimum of two participants should attend each meeting so they each have a professional partner at the meeting and, upon returning home, a colleague who had a common learning experience, thus making transfer of learning more likely. Prior to a meeting the participants should (1) decide which session(s) each will attend; (2) decide with whom they wish to meet to discuss mutual professional interests, and (3) call their colleagues' attention to important presentations, materials of interest, or people.

Competencies: 22.1–22.7, 23.1–23.15, 24.1–24.4.

Suggested Resource Material

For complete citations, see the Reference section at the end of this chapter. Also check the Annotated Bibliography for fuller description.

Aran, L., & Ben-David, J. (1968). Socialization and career patterns as determinants of productivity of medical researchers.

Bland, C. J., & Schmitz, C. C. (1986). Characteristics of the successful researcher and implications for faculty development.

McGaghie, W., & Frey, J. (1986). *Handbook for the academic physician.*

Mission statements, organizational charts, the tenure code, faculty handbook, constitution, and promotion guidelines from the participants' institutions.

Mission statements, organizations charts, funding programs, and funding history from various funding sources.

Mission statements, organizational chart, annual reports, membership guidelines, and publication lists from major professional and academic organizations.

Shils, E. A. (1983). *The academic ethic.*

Who faculty members are, and what they think. (1985). *Chronicle of Higher Education.*

502. MENTORSHIP WITH EXPERIENCED RESEARCHER
(One half-day per week for entire training period)

In a mentorship, the faculty participant serves as a research co-worker for a seasoned researcher. Mentors or advisors are critical to the complete development of researchers. Because of the importance of this experience, even traditional research training programs recommend that this relationship be more systematic.

Therefore, the mentorship should be as planned as possible. First, the mentor should be an experienced researcher and work in a field of interest to the participant. It helps if the mentor is interested in facilitating the development of the new researcher and able to spend meaningful time for at least 1 year with this person.

You will note that being a primary care physician or even physician researcher is not listed as a criteria, although it is preferred. Aran and Ben-David (1968) found that productivity in research increased more among those medical researchers whose resocialization took place in basic research than among those in a clinical research unit.

Second, both the mentor and participant should be familiar with the competencies expected to emerge as a result of the mentorship. Each needs to identify ways they can use the mentorship to achieve the expected competencies. It is best when the pair can build on the research interests of the participant, expertise of the mentor, and courses offered in the research domain.

In this curriculum, the research domain has an independent research project that calls for an advisor. You may therefore want to merge these two strategies. As a final suggestion, let us remind you that it may serve the participant best to work with more than one mentor. Both mentors and participants should realize that it is sometimes appropriate to change.

Competencies: 22.1–22.5, 22.7, 23.6–23.9, 24.1–24.4.

Rationale for Domain Design

In designing the curriculum for professional academic skills we asked two questions: What courses, activities, or overall structure would best help faculty to acquire these skills? How should these courses or activities be implemented?

To answer the first question, we unfortunately know very little about the best way to design a program to facilitate acquisition of the professional academic competencies because no institution (to our knowledge) does this, and the research we have to draw upon comes from other professions. In addition, this domain deals with changing people's attitudes and inculcating values as well as disseminating knowledge. Again, no writings specifically address ways to design such a program. Thus, to help us design the professional academic skill courses and strategies we turned to the research on occupational role socialization (e.g., Berkew & Hall, 1966; Brim & Wheeler, 1966), professional socialization (e.g., Jackson, 1970; Knopke & Anderson, 1981; Sherlock, 1967; Shuval & Adler, 1980; Singer, 1982), attitude development and social change (e.g., Lewin, 1958), and organization behavior (e.g., Van Maanen & Schein, 1979).

Professional socialization is typically accomplished through an informal, random, and lengthy process, although some professions (e.g., military, police) have fairly formal socialization programs, and corporations are quite sophisticated at quickly acculturating new employees. While the informal method has apparently been effective for most academic professionals, faculty in academic medicine have neither the mechanism nor the time for socialization to occur in this informal manner. Further, for members of newer disciplines such as family medicine or general internal medicine or for other less traditional faculty members such as women, minorities, and older or disabled persons, the informal socialization process has often been ineffective.

Recognizing this, professional organizations such as the Association of American Medical Colleges and Association of American Colleges have developed alternative socialization strategies for faculty in these groups. For example, the Committee on Women Historians writes, "The history professor operates in large measure by unwritten rules and historians who have had no coaching in these folkways often come to grief. The American Historical Association Committee on Women Historians decided that unwritten rules often lead to inequality and set out to reveal the most important rules and customs." Thus, for this and other reasons, we decided to make this portion of the curriculum both explicit and structured. In addition to being more efficient, using a structured approach is congruent with the recommendations of recent writers on academic socialization. For example, Corcoran and Clark (1986, p. 40) feel that "[socialization] . . . should be a more deliberate process." Conway and Glass (1978, p. 428) conclude similarly that "a thoughtfully planned socialization process could assure more success in the socialization of faculty."

The curriculum here, however, still relies on the two formats used most often in the informal socialization of academics: mentorship and peer group activities. We selected these strategies because they can be approached in a structured way. Also, "the typical strategy in graduate school socialization involves both collective processing (students in groups) and individual models (advisor guides students through their programs and dissertations individually)" (Corcoran & Clark, 1984, p. 141). These authors go on to assert that "peer relationships are an important part of socialization, for it is with peers that informal discussions, exchanges of aid and support, and friendships facilitate the learning that, in the present, tempers the 'ordeal' aspects of professional preparation and, in the future, prepares the student for collegial structures" (Corcoran & Clark, 1986, p. 35).

Mentorship, sometimes called sponsorship or role modeling, includes "advancement of a favored protégé, mentoring, and/or coaching a novice through the informal norms of the workplace and/or discipline" (Clark & Corcoran, 1986, p. 26). Mentorship has been found crucial for high achievement in many professions. For example, Oswold Hall's classic study of physicians in a Canadian community (Hall, 1949) established that novice physicians who were not sponsored by influential mentors enjoyed "friendly careers" but never achieved the higher status, income, or leadership of the protege group (Clark & Corcoran, 1986).

Bland and Schmitz (1986) reviewed studies on productive researchers and again found sponsorship to be a critical characteristic, one that distinguished productive researchers from other. Similarly, a study by Corcoran and Clark (1984) compared characteristics of highly active faculty with representative faculty and found that the highly active group reported more meaningful and enduring relationships with their advisor/mentors. Blackburn (1979) concludes that ". . . mentorship/sponsorship . . . is critical for . . . a productive career. Learning the informal network that supports productivity—the inner workings of professional associations and who the productive people are—is critical" (p. 25). Aran and Ben-David (1968) studied productive medical researchers and found that physician investigators learned certain connections and behaviors from working with established researchers. They reported that the productive researchers attached great importance to their continued contact with the scientists with whom they had worked during their research training.

Thus, our recommended curriculum follows the two traditional formats: group activity (in the form of a weekly seminar) and mentorship. Both are systematically structured.

Our second question in designing this curriculum concerned how these activities should be developed and implemented. The group seminar is collective, formal, and fixed; it is an ongoing, regular, and planned series of seminars—not a jumble of disparate talks. This design was based on a review of tactics in organizational socialization (Van Maanen

& Schein, 1979). "Tactics" refers to "the ways in which the experiences of individuals in transition from one role to another, are structured for them by the organization."

The typical tactics described are:

1. Collective vs. individual
2. Formal vs. informal
3. Sequential vs. variable
4. Fixed vs. variable
5. Serial vs. disjunctive
6. Investiture vs. divestiture

For this curriculum, the collective approach is used because it is more efficient and builds a collective sense of identity, solidarity, and loyalty within the cohort being socialized. A formal approach is used as it is most effective when acquisition of attitudes is a prime objective and when the socialization involves a complex set of attitudes and skills.

While some of the professional academic competencies are hierarchical, most are not. Thus, no specific sequence or timetable is set for the topics, although it is expected all competencies will be addressed in a planned fashion. This seminar design (collective, formal, fixed) is thought to produce a cohort with common knowledge and background and the ability to innovate and bring new ideas to their work.

As to the specific strategies to use in this seminar, the following guidelines were gleaned from consistent trends across these literatures. These guidelines then served as the basis for selecting strategies recommended for the professional seminar (501).

- Basic information, while insufficient alone, is essential for acquiring a new attitude, value, or social behavior. For example, knowing about the skills required to produce a painting increases appreciation for a masterpiece, and knowing the nutritional value, taste, and uses of an unfamiliar food increases the likelihood of it being incorporated into everyday eating habits (e.g., Lewin, 1958).
- Barriers to acquiring a new attitude or appreciation must be identified and addressed (e.g., Brim, 1968; Lewin, 1958; Rosow, 1974; Van Maanen & Schein, 1979; Wolansky & Oranu et al., 1978). Barriers include such things as information, beliefs, or behaviors that are inconsistent with the new attitude or behavior. For example, Lewin (1985) was unable to influence housewives' cooking habits by giving them information alone.

(His research was conducted during World War II when nutritionists developed educational programs on the benefits of using meat parts, such as sweetbreads, beef hearts, and kidneys, as a way to endure the meat shortages.) He was able to influence cooking habits by pairing information with discussion sessions that identified and countered unfounded beliefs about eating these meat parts. Interestingly, prior to these discussions, many of the housewives who declined to use these parts could not clearly explain why they were biased against them.

- Respected models who demonstrate the desired attitude or behavior are helpful (Block & Haan, 1971; Dager, Hines & Williams, 1976, Rice, 1983).
- Positive personal experience in using the new belief or behavior is essential (e.g., Mortimer & Simmons, 1978).
- Redundant strategies or repeated variations focused on the same competency may be necessary to affect a change in attitude or life-style (Taba, 1962).
- Teaching strategies most effective for changing attitudes include active methods such as small group discussion, simulations, role play, and debate (Deux & Wrightsman, 1984).

Annotated Bibliography

The references below were considered especially important to the content expert in defining and developing this domain. Therefore, they have been annotated, while other cited works have been included only in the Reference section. (For complete citations of these annotations and all other writings mentioned in this domain, turn to the Reference section at the end of this chapter).

Annotations can be very illuminating to readers for a number of reasons. First, they give readers who are not particularly familiar with the subject matter some important background information—a kind of "Cliff's Notes" to the curriculum content. Second, many of the annotations point to specific chapters or excerpts that may stimulate new ideas for teaching, or provide you with "quick-and-dirty" teaching materials. Third, they can help direct whatever further literature searches you may be planning in the area on your own.

Last, but not least, the discerning reader will learn much about the content expert's vision, perspective, or philosophic stance regarding his or her subject by reading these deliberately selected annotations. Perhaps even more than the prose in each rationale section, this bibliography may help you to see the subject matter as the content expert saw it and to understand why the domain is structured the way it is.

Blackburn, R. T. (1979). *Academic careers: Patterns and possibilities*

A noted researcher in career development in higher education and medicine, Blackburn presents nine conclusions about faculty productivity based on a thorough review of the literature. He prefaces these conclusions by first cautioning readers on the differences in expectations across institutional types, disciplines, and role functions. Expectations in productivity vary according to these groups. A second caveat, he explains, concerns the definition of "productivity." Most studies use the number of research articles published as a measure of productivity.

Given these statements, Blackburn summarizes a wide body of research on faculty productivity in the following statements:

1. The productivity of faculty over an entire career is predictable
2. The institution determines to a high degree a faculty member's productivity
3. Organizational factors influence faculty productivity
4. How time is structured affects productivity
5. Faculty interests and desire for different types of work change over the academic career
6. Age is not a predictor of productivity over a career path
7. Mentorship/sponsorship in the first year is critical for launching a productive career
8. Faculty productivity over a career is affected by security and by challenge
9. Rewards affect faculty performance, and intrinsic rewards dominate extrinsic ones

Some of these conclusions support our view that research productivity is dependent upon the organizational environment, an issue that need to be resolved in some primary care departments or hospital environments. Blackburn's other conclusions regarding age, career productivity, and mentorship are also interesting. Apparently a faculty member's age of first publication and age of receiving an advanced degree predict to an appreciable extent his or her career productivity. Over time, the discrepancy between productive and nonproductive people increases; prodigious researchers maintain their high level of output while less active faculty produce fewer and fewer studies. A significant trigger to early and continuous productivity is mentorship/sponsorship in the faculty member's first years. These findings also support the need for structured socialization for physician faculty.

Blackburn, R. T., & Fox, T. G. (1976). *The socialization of medical school faculty.*

In this study Blackburn and Fox compare the socialization processes of M.D.'s and Ph.D.'s into the faculty role. A five-part questionnaire (based on Sherlock and Morris's [1972] paradigm of professional development) was administered to 350 faculty at a midwestern university medical school. Data gathered included information on career backgrounds, attitudes toward issues within their school, and faculty's perceived and preferred organizational goals, characteristics, and managerial styles. Sample subjects were drawn from basic and clinical science departments; the ratio of M.D.'s to Ph.D.'s was 4 to 1 in the clinical sciences, and 1 to 4 in the basic sciences.

Sherlock and Morris's paradigm is a three-stage professional development model that links recruitment to socialization processes to professional outcomes. The survey results can be reported in terms of these three stages.

Recruitment.
Survey findings show that M.D.'s decide to become doctors early in life but decide to become academics relatively late. Ph.D.'s settle on an academic career in graduate or medical school, while M.D. faculty remain uncertain; at the very end of schooling only 52% of M.D. faculty knew they wanted an academic career. Whereas Ph.D.'s unconsciously socialized early in graduate school to academic role models, M.D.'s do not begin socializing to academe until they actually take their first faculty job.

Socialization Processes.
Blackburn and Fox postulate that the most critical of values for the academic is academic freedom. in this study, clinical faculty (predominantly M.D.'s) "perceived and feel academic freedom to be of less importance" than basic science faculty (predominantly Ph.D.'s). Clinical faculty did rate academic freedom highly, however. The authors conclude: "new values, academic ones, came late [to M.D. faculty] and had to come quickly" (p. 809).

In contrast, M.D.'s experience "high colleague acceptance" by the medical peers and mentors with whom they have trained. A substantial inbreeding of M.D. faculty occurs: over 70% of M.D.'s pursue their degree, internship, residency, and first faculty appointment at the same institution, whereas only 40% of Ph.D. faculty remain at one location.

Professional Outcomes.
In assessing occupational identity and commitment, the authors found

that M.D.'s maintain dual professional identify and never come to identify with the academic profession to the extent that basic science faculty do. A high turnover in M.D. faculty contrast with low Ph.D. turnover and occurs at earlier ages.

In their conclusions, the authors say that M.D. faculty need to be recruited and socialized earlier in their careers. In addition, recruitment should target research-oriented individuals. The medical school curriculum should be revised to include more research. And because faculty greatly influence the specialty students select, mentors should consciously socialize students to academic faculty roles.

Blackburn, R. T., & Fox, T. G. (1983). *Physicians' values and their career stage.*

In this study 241 practicing physicians in the northeastern United States were asked to rate the importance of 25 characteristics or features "of an ideal university medical school." A 50% response rate was obtained using a questionnaire whose 5-point scale ranged from 5 ("critical/essential") to 1 ("not really that important"). Through factor analysis the responses revealed seven factors (virtues of the medical center). These virtues are equated with the professional values held by the respondents. These factors are: academic, professional separatism, support, social welfare, research/specialization, status/prestige, and convenience.

The study's predominant outcome was the higher rating of practitioner values over academic values. Factor 2, professional separatism, received the highest overall mean (3.98). The items in this category deal with the referral of patients back to the original doctor, the prompt supply of information from the referring doctor, and the maintenance of good relationships between faculty and the community. In contrast, factor 1, academic, received the lowest overall mean (2.65). This factor contains items dealing with university activities. Receiving the lowest mean score of all 25 items was "opportunity for me to engage in research at the center" (1.84). Apparently, however, respondents do value the research that university faculty conduct, for they rated an item on this feature "important" (3.35).

Responses varied little between groups of physicians when categorized by specialty or training. The sample consisted of a rather homogeneous, well-educated, able, and highly socialized group of physicians; with the exception of surgery, values were equally distributed.

Differences were found between age cohorts, however. When responses were plotted by age (from 32 to 72 years old) in nine groups, five years apart, the professional separatism factor rose in importance among older faculty while the academic factor fell. The other factors of social welfare, research/specialization, support, status/prestige, and convenience fluctuated, generally increasing in importance after a period of sudden reversals in the 43 to 53 age groups.

Because the data are cross-sectional, not longitudinal, the authors cannot say whether these shifts are related to the career development or aging process or simply reflect the values of particular generations. Yet they strongly suspect the former. Their arguments reflect the work of Levinson and other adult development theorists (Levinson, Darrow, Klein, Levinson & McKee (1978). In this view, the new medical recruit is most altruistic; then, "his early academic enthusiasm fall off when these goals and values are not satisfied, when the business of establishing oneself and looking after one's financial security takes over" (p. 121). The fluctuations signal midlife transition, and academic values peak briefly in midlife and again in the oldest age group.

Of interest here is the value system of medical practitioners and how it may change during the course of a lifetime. One implication may be that new recruits, if they are to survive in academe, must be consciously supported and socialized in the early years of their career.

Bogdewic, S. (1986). *Advancement and promotion: Managing the individual career.*

Like other authors in this handbook, Bogdewic characterizes medical school departments as conflicted power structures with numerous and diverse programs, multiple funding sources, and unclear or contradictory goals. To advance in these settings, faculty must take charge of their careers early on. They do this first by choosing to work in professional settings that value their goals and skills and then by defining tasks, setting goals, and identifying resources. Scholastic ability as measured by tests and the prestige of the training institutions faculty attend do *not* predict survival in academic medicine. Longevity is determined, rather, by a faculty member's skill in managing his or her career.

Such management is the individual faculty member's responsibility and begins with values clarification:

> Certain skills, values and beliefs have to be present before a serious commitment can be made to a medical career. A similar process of self-examination should also precede the decision to become an academic physician. (p. 3)

To assist faculty with this self-examination, the author presents a sample of career questions that experienced faculty should advise junior colleagues to "ask of themselves" in considering an academic career.

Bogdewic then sketches out a three-stage career development model that corresponds to assistant, associate, and full professor statuses, respectively. The new faculty member is then advised on how to assess the match between personal aspirations and institutional expectations. An "activity analysis" is presented next; this exercise guides the documentation of faculty activities and time spent, along with their perceived value and degree of satisfaction.

The chapter goes on to address contracting and negotiating, two necessary strategies for planning and achieving career promotions. A prototypic PDC (Personal Development Contract) is described and presented, and suggestions for negotiating tasks and evaluations are offered. Bogdewic's "performance appraisal cycle" illustrates phases of career management and the processes of role negotiation, orientation, setting the professional development contract, formative reviews, gathering evaluation data, and annual evaluation. This is a very cogent chapter with sound practical advice for faculty administrators and faculty developers alike.

Cahn, S. M. (1986). *Saints and scamps: Ethics in academia.*

This book is a cross between Shils's *The Academic Ethic* and Sinderman's *The Joy of Science.* The author is a professor of philosophy who draws upon years of experience to provide ethical guidelines for teaching, scholarship, and academic personnel decisions. He begins with a brief overview of the significant autonomy that a faculty member enjoys. He agrees that this autonomy is essential for the role of a faculty member: the success of a democratic community depends in great part on the understanding and capability of its citizens, and so members of a free society need to ensure that those appointed to seek and communicate it to others are not interfered with on political, religious, or any other ground. This protection for faculty members has come to be known as, "academic freedom." This is the right of professionally qualified persons to discover, teach, and publish the truth as they see it within their fields of competence. (p. 5) He points out that this significant authority is paired with considerable professional responsibilities. The remainder of his book lays out these obligations and responsibilities because ". . .the first step toward discharging duties is to know what they are" (p. 7). He appropriately begins with the responsibility to teaching. It is teaching that is the one responsibility that all faculty members share, whether in 2-year colleges or highly research-oriented universities. He gracefully covers the major responsibilities of the teacher and the ethics underlying them.

The chapter on scholarship and service clearly delineates research obligations of a faculty member whose responsibilities are primarily teaching or who holds appointments at 2-year colleges from those whose major responsibilities are to prepare graduate students and advance knowledge. In addition to the scholarly tasks of a faculty member, here, as in teaching, the author describes the common underlying ethics. For example, he discusses plagiarism and authorship of articles. This chapter also talks about the community of scholars and the essential interrelatedness of academicians. Under *service* he refers to such things as departmental obligations and the writing of letters of recommendations for colleagues. The chapter on personnel decisions provides a good overview for new faculty who are not familiar with the search and appointment processes in universities.

The book is recent enough to reflect the affirmative action requirements that are in place at most universities and colleges. It is under personnel decisions that the author discusses tenure. He provides excellent examples of how the tenure system should work. Where tenure systems have not worked he puts blame not on the concept of a tenure system, but on the failure of faculty to carefully monitor who is awarded tenure and to appropriately dismiss incompetent members when necessary.

Corcoran, M., & Clark, S. M. (1984). *Professional socialization and contemporary career attitudes of three faculty generations.*

Corcoran and Clark are well known in higher education for their research in the areas of faculty and institutional vitality. Here they report results of an institutional case study in which differences in early socialization experiences and career attitudes of two faculty groups are compared. One group consists of 63 faculty members from diverse disciplines, judged to be "highly active" in research, teaching, and service. The other group consists of 66 tenured faculty randomly selected (and therefore "representative") but stratified by rank, field, and age to match the "highly active" faculty. The authors' premise is that socialization and career attitudes determine a faculty member's "vitality" (productivity).

Both *vitality* and *socialization* are, the authors admit, "vague," "poorly defined" terms, but rich in suggestive power. As emerging concepts they assist in theory construction by revealing complex variables, integrating disparate ideas, and leading to more specific concepts. As described by Maher (1982), *vitality* is "the capacity of the college or university to create and sustain the organizational strategies that support the continuing investment of energy by faculty and staff both in their own careers and in the realization of the institution's mission" (p. 3).

As described by organizational theorists, *socialization* is a process by which institutional and cultural values mold individual personality and behaviors. Together, socialization and vitality are the variables of interest to the institutional planner and faculty developer.

This particular study used an extended interview guide of 50 open-ended questions to probe differences between the highly active and representative faculty groups. Questions addressed their decision to enter academe, graduate school experience, personal career stages, work interests and preferences, productivity and success, morale, satisfaction, and future considerations.

Because this curriculum proposes to socialize medical faculty and to increase their research productivity, we find several of the study's outcomes interesting. First, 25% of the highly active group had parents who were educators, compared to only 10% of the representative group. Second, highly active faculty were originally attracted to research, whereas representative faculty were more attracted to teaching. Third, highly active faculty had many more socialization experiences (assistantships, etc.) than representative faculty. Finally, highly active faculty received more tangible help from advisors/mentors (e.g., positions offered, opportunities to collaborate, help in writing grants, contacts) after graduation than other faculty. In addition, the active group continued professional relationships with mentors and peers, whereas other faculty did not.

Dill, D. (1986). *Professional settings for the academic physician.*

More than perhaps any other single piece of literature, this chapter explains the importance of professional development skills for primary care faculty. Without the skills to clarify personal goals, to interpret conflicting demands of the environment, and to negotiate, faculty will neither prosper nor survive. The realities of an academic post frustrate many new faculty who bring with them "archtypal memories of the individual professional." In fact, Dill warns that "doctors who may be outstanding clinicians in private practice may be ineffective or unhappy in a medical school because they lack the skills and values required" (p. 3).

Several characteristics of academic medical centers make adjustment particularly difficult:

Complex roles. Although other professionals perform multiple tasks, only academic physicians perform them simultaneously. Research, education, and patient care can all occur during a single patient encounter. Each task serves a different constituency, makes its own demands, and imposes unique constraints.

Autonomy. In Weisbrod's (1978) study, 50% of the faculty said they were not responsible to anyone for their work. This tradition of autonomy works against new faculty who need support and feedback to learn their complex roles.

Reward system. As others have observed, the academic reward system is only loosely connected with the task system. Rewards come from different sources (money from patient care, promotion from research). This duality illustrates underlying conflicts in mission, values, and economic constraints.

Disorganization. As Dill says:

> Neither the administrative hierarchy, the work routine, nor the academic governance system has enough influence to integrate fully education, research, and patient care. Instead, integration is achieved through the loose and fluid form of a continual political process. (p. 6)

Departments. Last, in a majority of sites surveyed, department chairpersons were perceived as having more influence over medical school policies (education, research, patient care) than medical school deans. Additionally, the size of many departments requires that faculty assume administrative tasks early in their careers—even at the department chair level.

Learning to diagnose the ambiguity, conflict, and sources of personal stress is the first step new faculty need to acquire. Second, they need to become skilled negotiators and "creators of their own role." Third, they need to learn how to manage committees, and fourth, to initiate or participate in departmental organizational development.

Dill, D. (1986, April). *Local barriers and facilitators of research.*

Dill's purpose here is to review the evidence of contextual (i.e., organizational, environmental) factors on research productivity and to suggest how policy variables can be manipulated to enhance productivity. While pursuing these aims, the author illuminates much about the academic culture and implied value system pertinent to this domain.

Productivity is defined as publication counts and citations. The two primary contextual variables influencing productivity in both academic and research and development settings are institutional affiliation and organizational culture. Of the latter, leadership, selection of new faculty members, collegial and external communication, and workload are "moderating variables which help transform individual values into a reinforcing culture of research."

To develop and maintain a culture of research, the author makes several suggestions: (1) make sure that every appointed leader has demonstrated research abilities; (2) align the department/institutional evaluation and reward system with research values; (3) recruit new faculty from institutions that specialize in and socialize its graduates for research; and (4) support and provide faculty with access to relevant information channels inside and outside the institution.

Finally, the author argues for an integrated faculty body, where the tasks of research, teaching, and administration are shared by every member rather than a segregated department in which faculty work almost exclusively in research or teaching positions. Approximately 30% of faculty time should be devoted to research; flexible scheduling and leaves of absence allow for concentrated periods of investigation.

Houle, C. O. (1980). *Continued learning in the professions.*

Houle has given faculty developers a masterful synthesis of continuing education in the professions, drawn from research across 17 disciplines, including ministry, social work, dentistry, architecture, law, engineering, medicine, nursing, and others. His purpose is to compare how professionals "refresh their own knowledge. . . and build a sense of collective responsibility for society." In doing so he defines professionalism, stages of professional development, and the goals of lifelong learning. He catalogues the reason professionals seek out continued learning experiences and the correlates of such behavior. Finally, he offers recommendations for encouraging positive attitudes toward continued learning (both during formal training and after) and for setting up conducive environments and credible continuing education programs.

Houle's model of continuing education for professionals is nested within the larger training/socialization/continuing education process. Notably, the model begins with a period of general education, which may or may not include pretraining or entry requirements for formal training. Then, with the advent of specialized training, the novice is sequestered "psychologically if not physically" and heavily indoctrinated with the necessary knowledge, skills, and values of his or her future

profession. Once certified, the young graduaᵗᶜ is further supervised
and acculturated as he or she sets up practice at the chosen place of
employment. Continued education follows in various forms at various
times, as the professional prepares for a job shift or promotion, responds
to new technology, seeks recertification, develops new interests, or
suffers an identity crisis.

The prevailing notion of cor   .uing education is that it must serve
two functions: it must safeguard ᵗhe public from incompetence (and
the profession from a bad reputacion) and provide professionals with
opportunities for personal growth. The goals of continuing education
fall into two categories: that which professionals do to serve themselves,
and that which they do to serve the profession. As such, the goals
characterize the lifelong learner as someone who:

- continues to clarify the function(s) of the profession (mission,
  purpose, goals); "reality-tests" for change, evolution
- masters theoretical knowledge
- solves new problems; learns from every problem encountered
- updates and accesses a substantial body of knowledge
- strives for new personal dimensions of knowledge, skill, or sensitivity

Lifelong learners who constantly upgrade the profession do the following:

- improve/redesign formal training
- establish credentials and certification
- create a subculture: the lore, traditions, and so forth that
  characterize a profession
- enforce special rights and privileges of practitioners
- encourage public acceptance
- refine ethics of practice
- enforce penalties for malpractice
- seek alliances with other professions
- identify public relations needs and methods

Essentially, the author sees ongoing, self-directed learning as the trade-
mark of a mature professional, and ongoing, multifaceted education
as the goal of every mature profession. As such, these concepts resemble our notions of faculty development and faculty vitality and have
implications for several portions of the curriculum.

Houle's specific strategies to improve the institutional climate
include:

- Place as many educative features (library, lecture, release time, support systems) in the environment as resources allow.
- Systematically use a team approach within the organization; combining various specialists and backgrounds provides new dimensions to problem solving and new knowledge.
- Open up the decision-making process.
- Achieve goals but at every point "probe, learn, exchange ideas, open vistas."

Rice, R. E. (1983). *Being professional academically.*

"Faculty have different career anchors," the author says. There are different "career concept types" which in turn "require different kinds of situations in which to grow and develop—different sources of encouragement."

In addition, Rice says that the images professionals have of their roles are both necessary and important "socially constructed fictions." He then proceeds to outline the image or model of the academic professional that emerged during the "golden age" of higher education, the 1950's. The assumptions of this model are these:

- Research is the central professional endeavor and the focus of academic life.
- Quality is preserved in the academic profession through peer review and the maintenance of professional autonomy.
- The pursuit of knowledge is best organized according to discipline (and, as a consequence, disciplinary-based department structures).
- The distinctive task of the academic profession is the pursuit of cognitive truth.
- The pursuit of knowledge is for its own sake.
- Reputations are established through national and international professional associations.
- Professional rewards and mobility accrue to those who persistently accentuate their professions.

Although Rice goes on to explain how the above model is currently being challenged, particularly by faculty in particular types of institutions, the model embodies many of the foundation values of today's academic faculty. These are some of the values that may challenge, or come in conflict with, primary care faculty and practitioner values. This, therefore, has implications for developers who are interested in pursuing values clarification exercises with faculty.

Shils, E. A. (1983). *The academic ethic.*

This small (10-page) text enumerates the traditional values of academe, the purposes of a university, and the obligations of its professors. The ideal faculty member is described as a "custodian of knowledge," responsible for the generation and transmission of new knowledge and dedicated to the scientific method of inquiry. "Truth," as a rationally derived, objective entity, is the goal of both research and teaching. Intellectual integrity and freedom of inquiry are cherished beliefs.

An international committee of university professors authored this book. Considering the difficulties in writing by committee, particularly one made up of persons from other countries and cultures, the authors make many surprisingly strong and concrete statements. Although the text reads at times as dogma, it clearly presents not only an American but internationally held perception of academic beliefs and codes of conduct. This should be required reading for faculty members in highly research-oriented organizations. From the importance of research to the purpose of tenure to the evils of plagiarism, this text covers its ground well.

Sinderman, C. J. (1985). *The joy of science.*

Loosely described by the author as a collection of oral case histories gathered over a period of years, usually late at night, and recorded on cocktail napkins, this delightful, well-written book sums up the making of professional researchers in science. Its purpose is to trace the common career events and professional characteristics of successful scientists. It does so with insight and more rigor than the author (himself a researcher) implies.

In Part One Sinderman discusses the early socialization of researchers to the scientific method; the keys to managing a research team successfully; career transitions; and other challenges such as publishing and oral presentations. Part Two covers the "external" signs of success for mid-life researchers and the importance of networking and personal relations. What constitutes "good science" is heartily discussed, along with "controversies, frauds, burn-out, fade-out, guaranteed losers," and other topics. Women in science receive a special chapter, as do aging scientists.

The author's honesty about the virtues and vices of academe is refreshing. His good humor makes this an enjoyable book to read. For readers new to academe and the research ethic, it provides many good profiles of successful academic professionals and insights on why they do what they do.

Wheeler, D., & Creswell, J. (1985). *Developing faculty as researchers.*

This paper is the product of an impressive literature review in the areas of the sociology of science and faculty career development. The purpose of the review was to identify the predictive correlates of high research performance and their context within the stages of faculty careers so that appropriate faculty development strategies for developing researchers could be devised.

"Research productivity" is defined as a range of scholarly activities that culminate in publishing and is measured in terms of publication and citation counts. Faculty development is defined as any set of "program activities, practices, and strategies that aim both to maintain and to improve the professional competence of individual faculty members" (Mathis, 1982, p. 646). The authors conducted their search for correlates and organized them in their presentation according to three categories.

Category one contains individual person variables, such as IQ, motivation, personality, age, and gender. Category two contains variables relating to the educational organizations influencing faculty's training and productivity, such as doctoral program, sponsorship by mentors, colleagues, resources, and assignment. Category three variables are measures of the individual/environment interaction, such as early productivity, research orientation, discipline differences, and stress.

The career stage model used was developed by Mathis (1979) and consists of four stages: (1) graduate preparation, (2) initial years as faculty, (3) middle and later years, and (4) retirement and beyond. The authors suggest that the beginning phases of each of the above career stages are sensitive periods when faculty may be most in need of, or receptive to, faculty development efforts.

For our purposes, correlates from the organizational and individual/environmental categories are the most relevant. These are variables that faculty development can do something about, unlike gender or IQ. They also affect research productivity and were usually overlooked in past training efforts. Significant findings include the following:

- Graduate school mentors directly influence the predoctoral and early publication efforts of young scholars for 3 to 6 years postgraduation. Sponsorship includes financial and placement support, publication and sponsored research support, first job placement, collaboration, and emotional support.
- The prestige of the training (doctoral) institution and the prestige of the employing institution both shape and stimulate individual research performance.
- Early habits of publishing and the number of publications in the first 1 to 5 years predict lifetime productivity.
- As a group, faculty interest in research peaks at age 30, then declines as less research-oriented faculty turn to teaching and administration. "The percentage of 'exclusive teachers' doubles, and 'strong researchers' halves between the ages of 35–56" (p. 7).
- Highly productive scholars maintain frequent contact with colleagues within and outside their institution.
- The workplace exercises a strong influence on research productivity in terms of reinforcement and rewards. Attitudes of both administrators and colleagues affect performance.
- Faculty who work on simultaneous topics and establish continuous lines of research (lasting 5 years or more) publish more than those who do not.

The authors conclude with various recommendations about mentoring, role assignments, colleagues, and departmental attitudes. The intangible "respect and support for research" can be translated into sincere interest, sympathy, and praise for what researchers are doing, and adequate support services.

References

Aran, L., & Ben-David, J. B. (1968). Socialization and career patterns as determinants of productivity of medical researchers. *Health and Social Behavior, 9*(1), 3–15.

Berkew, D. E., & Hall, D. T. (1966). The socialization of managers: Effects of expectation on performance. *Administrative Science Quarterly, 11,* 207–223.

Blackburn, R. T. (1979). Academic careers: Patterns and possibilities. *Current Issues in Higher Education, 2,* 25–27.

Blackburn, R. T., & Fox, T. G. (1976). The socialization of medical school faculty. *Journal of Medical Education, 51,* 806–817.

Blackburn, R. T., & Fox, T. G. (1983). Physicians' values and their career stage. *Journal of Vocational Behavior, 22,* 159–173.

Bland, C. J., Hitchcock, M., Anderson, W., & Stritter, F. T. (1986, March). *Study of graduates of family medicine faculty development fellowship programs.* Final report of the Society of Teachers of Family Medicine Task Force on Faculty Development. Co-funded by the Robert Wood Johnson Foundation and the Division of Medicine, HRSA Contract #84 592(p). Minneapolis: University of Minnesota.

Bland, C. J., Hitchcock, M. A., Anderson, W. A., & Stritter, F. T. (1987, August). Faculty development fellowship programs in family medicine. *Journal of Medical Education, 62*(8), 632–641.

Bland, C. J., & Schmitz, C. C. (1986). Characteristics of the successful researcher and implications for faculty development. *Journal of Medical Education, 61,* 22–31.

Block, J., & Haan, N. (1971). *Lives through time.* Berkeley, CA: Bancroft.

Bogdewic, S. (1986). Advancement and promotion: Managing the individual career (pp. 22–36). In W. C. McGaghie & J. J. Frey (Eds.), *Handbook for the academic physician.* New York: Springer-Verlag.

Brim, O. G., Jr. (1968). Adult socialization. In J. Clausen (Ed.), *Socialization and society.* Boston: Little, Brown & Company.

Brim, O. G., & Wheeler, S. (1966). *Socialization after childhood: Two essays.* New York: John Wiley.

Bucher, R., & Stelling, J. G. (1977). *Becoming professional.* Beverly Hills, CA: Sage Publications.

Caffrey, J. (1969). Predictions for higher education in the 1970's. In J. Caffrey (Ed.), *The future academic community.* Washington, DC: American Council on Education.

Cahn, S. M. (1986). *Saints and scamps: Ethics in academia.* Totoway, NJ: Rowman & Littlefield.

Cameron, S. W., & Blackburn, R. T. (1981). Sponsorship and academic career success. *Journal of Higher Education, 52*(4), 369–377.

Clark, S., & Corcoran, M. (1986). Perspectives on the professional socialization of women faculty. *Higher Education, 57*(1), 20–43.

Conway, M. E., & Glass, L. K. (1978). Socialization for survival in the academic world. *Nursing Outlook, 26*(7), 424–429.

Corcoran, M., & Clark, S. M. (1984). Professional socialization and contemporary career attitudes of three faculty generations. *Research in Higher Education, 20*(2), 131–153.

Creswell, J. (1985). *Faculty research performance: Lessons from the sciences and the social sciences.* ASHE/ERIC Higher Education Research Report No. 4. Washington, DC: Association for the Study of Higher Education.

Dager, E. Z., Hines, D., & Williams, J. B. (1976). *Social identification, social influences and value transmission.* Paper presented at the 71st Annual Meeting of the American Sociological Association, New York, NY.

David, A. K. (1981). Fellows in family medicine—1979–1980. *Family Medicine, 13,* 8–11.

Deux, K., & Wrightsman, L. S. (1984). Theories of attitude change. *Social psychology in the 80's.* Monterey, CA: Brooks/Cole.

Dill, D. (1986a, April). *Local barriers and facilitators of research.* Paper presented at the meeting of the American Educational Research Association, San Francisco. CA.

Dill, D. (1986b). Professional settings for the academic physician. In W. C. McGaghie & J. J. Frey (Eds.), *Handbook for the academic physician* (pp. 3–10). New York: Springer-Verlag.

Dubin, R. (Ed.). (1976). *Handbook of work, organization, and society.* Chicago: Rand McNally College.

Hagstrom, W. O. (1965). *The scientific community.* New York: Basic Books.

Hall, O. (1949). Types of medical careers. *American Sociology, 155,* 243–253.

Hill, R., & Aldous, J. (1969). Socialization for marriage and parenthood (pp. 885–950). In D. Gaslin (Ed.), *Handbook of socialization: Theory and research.* Chicago: Rand McNally.

Houle, C. O. (1980). *Continued learning in the professions.* San Francisco: Jossey-Bass.

Jackson, J. A. (Ed.). (1970). *Professions and professionalization.* Cambridge, England: Cambridge University Press.

Knopke, H. J., & Anderson, R. L. (1981). Academic development in family medicine. *Family Practice, 12*(3), 483–499.

Levinson, D. J., Darrow, C. N., Klein, E. B., Levinson, M. H., & McKee, B (1978). *The seasons of a man's life.* New York: Knopf.

Lewin, K. (1958). Group decision and social change. In E. E. Macoby, T. M. Newcomb, & E. L. Hartley (Eds.), *Readings in social psychology.* New York: Henry Holt.

Maher, T. H. (1982). Institutional vitality in higher education. AAHE & ERIC Research Currents, *AAHE Bulletin, 34*(10), 3–6.

McGaghie, W., & Frey, J. (1986). *Handbook for the academic physician.* New York: Springer-Verlag.

Moore, W. E. (1969). Occupational socialization. In D. Gaslin (Ed.), *Handbook of socialization: Theory and research.* Chicago: Rand McNally.

Mortimer, J. T., & Simmons, R. F. (1978). Adult socialization. *Annual Review of Sociology, 4,* 421–454.

Neugarten, B. L (Ed.). (1968). *Middle age and aging: A reader in social psychology.* Chicago: University of Chicago Press.

Nyre, G. F., & Reilly, K. C. (1979). *Professional education in the eighties: Challenges and responses.* AAHE/ERIC Higher Education Research Report No. 8. Washington, DC: American Association for Higher Education.

Pelz, D. C., & Andrews, F. M. (1966). *Scientists in organizations: Productive climates for research and development.* New York: John Wiley.

Rice, R. E. (1983, April). Being professional academically. In D. T. Bedsole (Ed.), *Critical aspects of faculty development programs.* Proceedings of the Invitational Seminar on Faculty Development, Sherman, TX. Eric ED 238 387.

Rosow, I. (1974). *Socialization to old age.* Berkeley: University of California Press.

Sherlock, B. J. (1967, September). *Socialization cycle in professional schools.* Paper presented at meeting of the American Sociological Association, San Francisco, CA.

Sherlock, B. J., & Morris, R. T. (1972). *Becoming a dentist.* Springfield, IL: Charles C Thomas.

Shils, A. (1983). *The academic ethic.* Report of a Study Group of the International Council on the Future of the University. Chicago: University of Chicago Press.

Shuval, J. T., & Adler, I. (1980). The role of models in professional socialization. *Social Science and Medicine, 14A*(1), 5–14.

Sinderman, C. J. (1985). *The joy of science.* New York: Plenum Press.

Singer, D. L. (1982). Professional socialization and adult development in graduate professional education. *New Directions for Experiential Learning, 16,* 45–63.

Taba, H. (1962). *Curriculum development.* New York: Harcourt, Brace & World.

Van Maanen, J., & Schein, E. H. (1979). Toward a theory of organization socialization. *Research Organizational Behavior, 1,* 209–264.

Weisbord, M. R. (1978). Why organization development hasn't worked (so far) in medical centers. In: *Organizational diagnosis: A workbook of theory and practice.* M. R. Weisbord (Ed.), Reading, MA: Addison-Wesley, 168–180.

Wheeler, D., & Creswell, J. (1985, March). *Developing faculty as researchers.* Paper presented at the Annual Meeting of the Association for the Study of Higher Education, Chicago, IL.

Who faculty members are, and what they think. (1985, December 18). *Chronicle of Higher Education, 21,* 2–4.

Wolansky, W. D., & Oranu, R. (1978). Evaluation, confusion, and alternatives in our struggle for excellence. *College Student Journal, 12*(1), 40–47.

CHAPTER **8**

Curriculum Implementation Models

This chapter addresses questions of implementation. Given the content domains of professional academic skills, research, education, administration and written communication, given the goals and specific competencies, suggested courses, activities, and resource materials for each of these domains, how may they be organized in practical fashion for academic physician learners?

A crucial step in curriculum design, of course, is to identify the audience for whom instruction is intended and then identify its specific learning needs. Thus, the first step in building a faculty development program is to identify the likely participants and the specific skills they need to function optimally in their faculty roles. Armed with this list of competencies, or training objectives, the second step is to assemble and implement strategies that will accomplish the training objectives. You can select or modify the strategies described in this book, draw on other resources at your local university, or completely design your own strategies. Most likely, you will do a combination of the above. The third step is to sequence these strategies as logically as possible given practical constraints such as courses that are offered only during certain times of the year, availability of training staff, availability of participants, and so on.

To illustrate a range of implementation strategies, we have designed four faculty development models based on the requisite competencies for the four types of faculty described in Chapter 1 (A)—Introduction. Recall that the four types are: (1) Tenure-track in research-oriented universities, (2) tenure-track in comprehensive universities and some community settings, (3) non-tenure-track in universities or community settings, and (4) preceptor faculty. The distinction between research-oriented universities and comprehensive universities is that the missions of research, teaching, and service are more equally addressed in comprehensive universities.

Each model program is designed to address *all* the requisite competencies of one faculty type. In the case where program participants are experienced faculty members, a needs assessment should be conducted to identify the particular skills that remain to be learned, and therefore which strategies to emphasize or delete.

These models, then, are suggested plans for combining goals, competencies, and courses into programs for the four faculty types in primary care. In terms of amount of content covered, level of expectation, and content emphasis, they range from 2-day institutes to 3-year fellowships. In terms of delivery location, they include programs delivered entirely "off-site" (at a regional faculty development center or university), programs delivered entirely "on-site" (at participating faculty members' home institutions), and programs involving both on-site and off-site locations for varying periods of time.

Two general biases guided the development of these implementation plans. First, we consider faculty development a professional endeavor, one that requires substantial planning, expert personnel in several areas and time. A lot can go wrong! Whether the program is built for a single faculty type or all four, whether it consists of 1-day workshops or 3-year residential training, faculty development should be carefully planned. Few departments or residency programs, we believe, have the critical resources necessary to engineer a comprehensive, structured program for more than one type of faculty member. (This belief is supported by site visits, surveys, experience, and information gained through professional networking.) For this reason, the two residential fellowship plans take place at major universities. The remaining plans, targeted for existing faculty, emphasize an off-site approach to training. The amount of time spent off-site varies, but each plan relies on an external component to some extent. Off-site periods range from 3 months (24-month on/off-site plan) to 2-day institutes. (Institutes may, of course, be held on-site , but even these would probably bring in some external consultants.)

In developing the on- and off-site plans we tried to capitalize on the advantages of each setting; we aimed to make the most appropriate use of the respective resources. Thus, we looked to the off-site component for content expertise in research and to the home site for opportunities to apply knowledge or do projects (e.g., conduct an organizational diagnosis, develop a course). We looked to the off-site component for greatest exposure to academic values and activities, and to the home site for the retention of clinical skills and content.

In capitalizing on the strengths of home and off-site settings, we make a further assumption that the curricula in the off-site programs are of high quality. Because these programs can be run from year to year, evaluated and revised systematically, and staffed with faculty development professionals with significant time commitments, off-site programs have the ability to perfect their curriculum over time. This assumption applies to 2-day institutes as well as to longer plans. These features of stability and professionalism would appear to give clear advantage to off-site programs, especially if local programs are developed by inexperienced developers, are run only once, and are never (or minimally) evaluated.

The second bias reflected in the implementation plans presented here is our decision to *not* design on-site 9- and 12-month training periods (see Appendix). Because of the relatively lower success of nine- and 12-month fellowships found in the Study of Graduates and the Study of Federally Funded Faculty Development Programs (Bland, Hitchcock, Anderson & Stritter, 1987), we feel that longer on-site training formats are necessary for any curriculum that includes research.

Table 8.1 summarizes the primary features of each implementation plan. In the text that follows, we elaborate on each plan's intended audience(s), its curriculum emphasis, and other special characteristics. We also list each plan's advantages and disadvantages to developers and to participants. The actual configuration of courses for each implementation plan is presented graphically by accompanying "maps" (diagrams). These maps indicate how the courses described in the five individual domain sections may be integrated and sequenced during the time allotted. Approximately 522 hours of instruction time are identified for the 2-year fellowship, 424 for the 24-month home off-site plan, 168 for the 12-month home off-site plan, and 16 hours for the 2-day institutes. Because the 3-year fellowship depends heavily on university course work, it is difficult to estimate the number of instructional hours. Still, this plan is clearly the most intensive.

Three-Year Fellowship

Description

This plan is designed for physicians who are or expect to be full-time, tenured faculty in a research-oriented university. Except for the research

TABLE 8.1 Highlights of Five Implementation Plans

Three-Year Fellowship
- Tenure-track, research university
- Residency graduates
- National sites
- Produces career researchers in specialized areas
- Five domains; extensive coverage but research given greatest priority
- Extended mentor time for socialization to academe
- 20% clinical time
- Program likely leads to master's-level research degree

Two-Year Fellowship
- Tenure-track, comprehensive university
- Residency graduates
- Regional or national sites
- Five domains, extensive coverage
- Considerable opportunity for socialization to academe
- Produces full-time "research generalist"
- 30% clinical time
- May result in master's-level research degree

24-Month Home/Off-Site
- Tenure-track, teaching university or community setting
- New and existing faculty
- Six periods away from home at regional sites
- Five domains; extensive coverage
- Home-base program bears some training responsibility: project supervising, mentoring, independent study
- Produces full-time "faculty generalist" (research and teach)

12-Month Home/Off-Site
- Non-tenure-track, both settings
- New and existing faculty
- Four periods away from home at regional sites
- Five domains; coverage emphasizes teaching and administration
- Home-base program bears training responsibility for projects, practicums
- Produces full- or part-time "teaching generalist"

2-Day Institutes
- Preceptors and non-tenure-track, all settings
- New and existing faculty
- Three domains: Education, Research, and Administration
- Participants elect one domain per institute
- No ongoing project or practicum
- Few home-base responsibilities
- Full- or part-time "practice generalist"

---

component, the 3-year fellowship curriculum is essentially identical to the 2-year fellowship in terms of content and strategies. Participants in both fellowships experience the same education, administration, written communication, and professional socialization activities. In the 3-year model, however, participants acquire the research competencies by enrolling in a formal university degree program that provides a sequence of structured research courses and an advising system. Participation in the 3-year fellowship should lead to a master's degree in a research-related field such as epidemiology, sociology, or anthropology.

Because of this model's emphasis on structured research courses and research mentors, it can realistically be instituted only at major research universities with rich resources in terms of faculty and support services. This plan recommends the least amount of clinical time of the five implementation plans presented—20%. This allotment closely resembles clinical time recommended in other programs designed to train researchers, such as the NIH research training programs or the Robert Wood Johnson Foundation Clinical Scholars program.

Readers should note that for the other implementation plans the courses and activities described in this book (and listed on the implementation maps) have been specifically designed around the requisite competencies. For the research domain in this model, readers will have to determine whether existing degree programs and courses at the university address the requisite research competencies or not. Likely places to locate appropriate degree programs and courses are schools of public health, colleges of education, and departments of sociology or environmental health. It is hazardous to presume, however, that any course entitled "Research Design," for example, covers the required research design competencies for a tenure-track faculty member in a research-oriented university. A careful review of course curricula and activities is required before placing existing courses into the faculty development curriculum. Even better, a consultation with course professors or observation of classes is highly recommended.

Advantages and Disadvantages of the Three-Year Fellowship Model

There are tradeoffs in whichever implementation model is used, both for the participant and his or her home-base institution (provided the participant is currently employed as a faculty member). The most obvious advantage of the 3-year model is that it provides faculty with sufficient research training. Bland and Schmitz reported a study conducted by NIH in 1986 that revealed only 14 percent of the physician investigators with 19 to 30 months of research training subsequently appeared in and received NIH grants. Success rates for fellows with 31–42 months of training rose to 25 percent; after 43 months the success rate was 33 percent. . . Research projects are of course, funded by other sources, but the correlation between time spent in training and successful competition for NIH funds remains impressive. (1986, p. 28)

The most obvious drawbacks are expense, demands on faculty participants in terms of commitment, and caliber of resources needed within the university. Given the investment that is required, it is essential that an appropriate match be made between the learners and the actual program that is planned.

Whichever plan is considered, the engagement of capable staff is a prerequisite. Thus, each of the five models, "able staff" is a potential advantage and lack of able staff a potential disadvantage to consider.

Advantages

- comprehensive training in all domains
- maximum access to academic mentors
- provides socialization in an academic setting
- most likely to train faculty who can eventually function as academic mentors for others
- resource-rich environment for learning
- longest training program is most realistic for research development

Disadvantages

- most expensive in terms of time and money
- few settings have all the necessary resources to offer this model
- a limited number of learners can be trained in this way
- clinical time is very limited
- costly delay to the beginning of a faculty member's paid career
- probably not feasible for existing faculty

Implementation Map

Figure 8.1 shows how courses for the 3-year fellowship can be integrated and sequenced over a 36-month period. Except for research courses to be identified by the planner at the university, the course numbers and tables listed on the diagram match those described earlier in the five content domains.

Two-year Fellowship

Description

The 2-year fellowship is the second-longest training model of the five suggested plans. Like the 3-year fellowship, it consists of intensive, residential training that covers all five content domains thoroughly. The most likely candidate for this plan is the recent medical residency graduate who has not yet settled in a department but is clearly working toward a full-time, tenure-track position at a comprehensive university. It may also suit the physician who has been in full-time practice and wishes to make a career shift into a full-time academic position with research responsibilities. While the curriculum would reasonably benefit existing faculty, faculty who are non-tenure-track would find this less appealing.

Both the 2- and 3-year fellowships adopt a preparatory approach to education. They deliberately sequester fellows from much of the administrative and patient care duties of faculty life and provide ample opportunities for academic socialization through weekly professional development seminars and collaboration with mentors. A research project is planned and conducted with the help of the mentor and other consultants. Standard course work in statistics, research design, and other subjects pertinent to the fellow's research area are specially designed or arranged on campus. Bimonthly consultations with a writing consultant are expected. Practica in education and administration are arranged in conjunction with coursework. As much as possible, the curriculum is organized so that offerings in one domain complement those in another. The 2-year fellowship enables physician faculty to function on a high, well-rounded level. Their skills will enable them to plan curricula, teach, manage committees and staff, conduct research, and write.

Advantages and Disadvantages of the Two-Year Fellowship Model

This plan involves some of the same advantages and disadvantages as the 3-year fellowship, but to lesser degrees. Its greatest disadvantage (compared to the 3-year fellowship) is that it is difficult for faculty

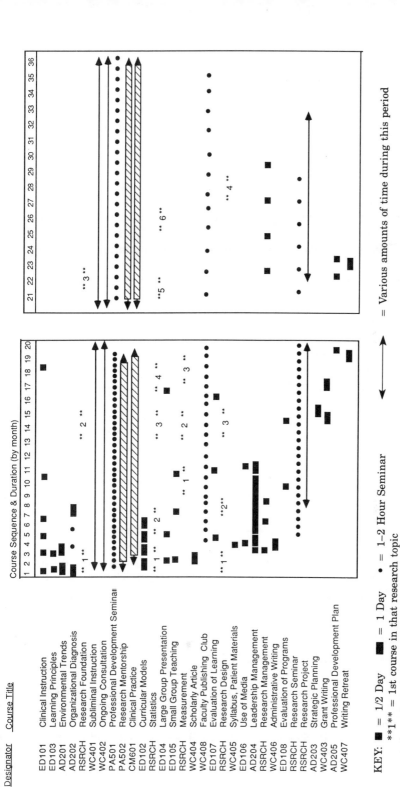

FIGURE 8.1 Three-year fellowship (primary participant: tenure-track, research university).

to complete both the necessary course work and an actual research study within 2 years. Its greatest asset (compared to the 3-year fellowship) is that it is 1 year shorter and makes fewer demands, yet still prepares faculty well for many institutional settings.

Advantages

- provides extensive training in all five domains
- provides opportunity for socialization to academe
- 2-year training has proven effective in training many primary care researchers
- provides opportunity for networking with training peers and staff
- likely to provide faculty who can function as academic mentors for others

Disadvantages

- very expensive
- requires a setting with many resources, e.g., clinic, computer, statistical services, libraries, teaching other practice opportunities
- requires significant time from participants and staff
- may not reserve enough clinical time for some fellows
- delays entry of fellows into faculty positions
- probably not feasible for many existing faculty
- probably not enough time to acquire necessary research skills and socialization to succeed in a research-oriented university

Implementation Map

Figure 8.2 shows how courses and other activities may be organized, integrated, and sequenced over a 24-month period. The course numbers and titles listed on the map match those described earlier in each of the respective domains.

24-Month Home/Off-Site Plan

This program is intended for existing or new full-time, tenure-track faculty either in community-based programs or teaching universities that are somewhat oriented to research. The curriculum is broad in scope, covering all five domains, and reflects a modified preparatory approach. The curriculum also allows full-time

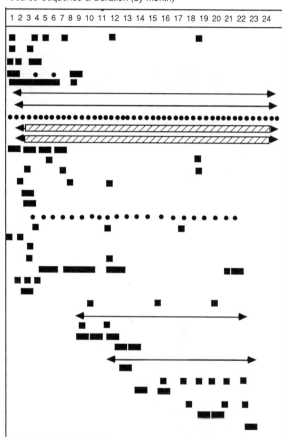

Course Sequence & Duration (by month)

Designator	Course Title
ED101	Clinical Instruction
ED103	Learning Principles
AD201	Environmental Trends
AD202	Organizational Diagnosis
RS301	Introduction to Research
WC401	Subliminal Instruction
WC402	Ongoing Consultation
PA501	Professional Development Seminar
PA502	Research Mentorship
CM601	Clinical Practice
ED102	Curricular Models
RS302	Assessing Research Literature
ED104	Large Group Presentation
ED105	Small Group Teaching
RS303	Using a Library
WC404	Scholarly Article
WC408	Faculty Publishing Club
ED107	Evaluation of Learning
RS304	Integrated Research Review
WC405	Syllabus, Patient Materials
ED106	Use of Media
AD204	Leadership Management
RS305	Research Planning
WC406	Administrative Writing
ED108	Evaluation of Programs
RS309	Research Project
RS306	Data Management
RS308	Advanced Methods
RS307	Introduction to Statistics
RS311	Formal Coursework
AD203	Strategic Planning
RS310	Research Seminar
WC403	Grant Writing
AD205	Professional Development Plan
WC407	Writing Retreat
RS312	Research Conference

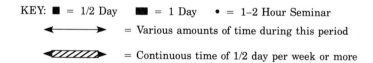

KEY: ■ = 1/2 Day   ■■ = 1 Day   • = 1–2 Hour Seminar

⟵⟶ = Various amounts of time during this period

⟸▨▨▨⟹ = Continuous time of 1/2 day per week or more

FIGURE 8.2 Two-year fellowship model (primary participant: tenure-track, comprehensive university).

faculty to integrate work experience with serious professional training in a manner that meets their individual interests. Participants who complete this plan would be well trained as "faculty generalists," able to teach, administer programs, and conduct a modest number of research studies over time.

The major portion of the participant's time is spent at his or her home site. Most of the structured course activities, however, are conducted by faculty developers at a regional or national training site during six periods that participants spend away from their department. These periods are scheduled over 2 years and are 1 month, 2 weeks, and one-and-one-half weeks long (see Figure 8.3). In between these off-site periods, faculty participants are expected to prepare assignments, study, work on individual projects, and meet with editors, consultants, and mentors, as well as contribute to their department's activities (e.g., patient care, administration). For this reason, the home-base department bears a considerable responsibility for their faculty's training in this plan. Before faculty enroll in home off-site programs, department or residency leaders would have to agree to support the program's goals and contribute to the faculty member's training.

Advantages and Disadvantages of the 24-Month Home/Off-Site Plan

Plans that incorporate home-based applications training with intensive periods off-site in regional or national faculty development centers can achieve the best of both worlds (provided they are well done), particularly for the generalist faculty member with moderate expectations in research. The primary disadvantages stem from poor coordination between home-base and off-site training objectives and from difficulties participants may have with bringing back to the department what was learned during training.

Advantages

- intensive training periods with professionals and peers across the country
- allows for immediate application of new skills to real work at home
- provides some opportunity to build links with training peers and staff and networks for the future
- provides broad training in all areas
- logistically feasible for existing faculty

- contributes to home setting via research (and other) projects

Disadvantages

- fairly expensive
- requires immense home support and resources
- effectiveness depends on the integration of resources and cooperation between training and home sites
- may have insufficient contact hours with off-site staff
- probably no home-base mentor or editor
- may disrupt ongoing home site and family responsibilities
- requires significant travel

Implementation Maps

Figure 8.3 illustrates how courses and other activities may be sequenced and integrated for the 24-month home/off-site plan. The course numbers and titles listed on the map match those described earlier in each respective domain.

12-Month Home/Off-Site Plan

Description

This plan is best suited for the full-time, non-tenure-track faculty member in either the university or community setting. Likely candidates for this plan are new or existing faculty who wish to improve their teaching and administrative skills. Although the five domains are still covered, course time in research, written communication, and professional academic skills is greatly reduced and modified in terms of mastery levels. The emphasis in these courses also shifts. For example, in Research the ability to access and interpret literature is stressed, not research design or management. In Written Communication, grant writing, administrative writing, and educational materials are taught, not scholarly writing for medical journals. In Professional Academic Skills, understanding university traditions (the academic system) and recognizing value differences are taught, but mentorships are not assigned. These domains might, in fact, be considered optional, a reflection of the continuing medical education influence in this model.

Most of the participant's time is spent in his or her home department. Four off-site periods are scheduled (2 weeks, one-and-one-half

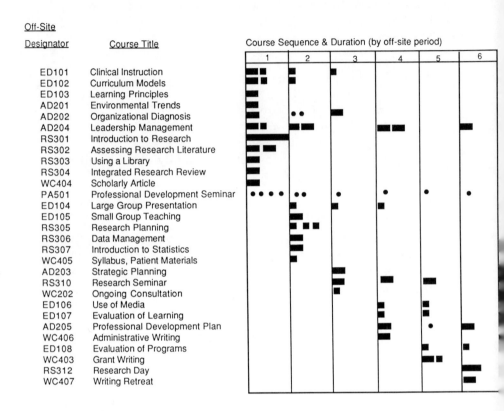

FIGURE 8.3 24-month home/off-site model (primary participant: tenure-track, community setting or teaching university).

weeks, and 1 week in length) over the course of a year. Faculty at national or regional training centers teach the specified course activities. The home-base department also bears some responsibility for their faculty members' training. Specifically, they need to provide a small amount of release time for study and projects related to the participant's course work.

Although this plan does not terminate in a graduate degree, it should carry some rewards for recognition of participation. A participant from this program would be well trained in clinical teaching and administration and better acclimated to the academic medical environment.

Advantages

- provides some opportunity to interact with training peers and staff for future networking
- provides sufficient training in some areas, introductory training in others
- has potential for helping faculty to develop a mentor at home
- logistically feasible for existing faculty
- allows for immediate application of new skills to real work at home
- requires minimal time away from home
- contributes to home setting via participant projects

Disadvantages

- requires significant expenditures
- requires considerable home support and resources
- insufficient training time for some areas
- effectiveness depends on the integration of activities and coordination between training and home site
- may provide insufficient contact hours with off-site staff
- no home-site mentor or editor
- has discontinuous learning sessions with staff and training peers
- may disrupt family responsibilities
- may disrupt some collegial relationships or responsibilities at home
- requires significant travel

Implementation Map

Figure 8.4 shows how courses and other activities may be integrated

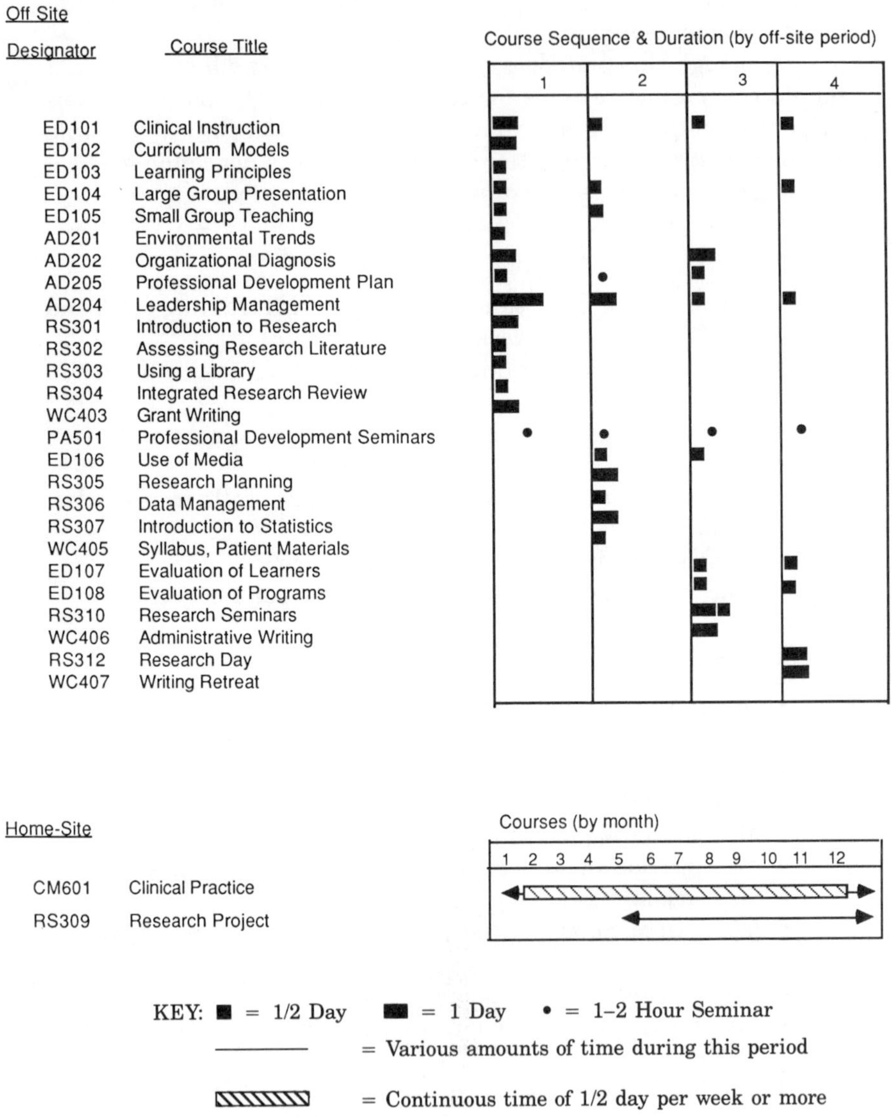

Off Site

Designator	Course Title	Course Sequence & Duration (by off-site period)			
		1	2	3	4
ED101	Clinical Instruction				
ED102	Curriculum Models				
ED103	Learning Principles				
ED104	Large Group Presentation				
ED105	Small Group Teaching				
AD201	Environmental Trends				
AD202	Organizational Diagnosis				
AD205	Professional Development Plan				
AD204	Leadership Management				
RS301	Introduction to Research				
RS302	Assessing Research Literature				
RS303	Using a Library				
RS304	Integrated Research Review				
WC403	Grant Writing				
PA501	Professional Development Seminars				
ED106	Use of Media				
RS305	Research Planning				
RS306	Data Management				
RS307	Introduction to Statistics				
WC405	Syllabus, Patient Materials				
ED107	Evaluation of Learners				
ED108	Evaluation of Programs				
RS310	Research Seminars				
WC406	Administrative Writing				
RS312	Research Day				
WC407	Writing Retreat				

Home-Site

Courses (by month)

		1 2 3 4 5 6 7 8 9 10 11 12
CM601	Clinical Practice	
RS309	Research Project	

KEY: ■ = 1/2 Day ▬ = 1 Day • = 1–2 Hour Seminar

――――― = Various amounts of time during this period

▨▨▨▨ = Continuous time of 1/2 day per week or more

FIGURE 8.4 12-month home/off-site model (primary participant: non-tenure-track, any setting).

and sequenced over a 12-month period. The course numbers and titles listed on the map match those described earlier in each of the respective domains.

Two-Day Institutes

Description

These intense 48-hour training sessions cover three domains (Education, Administration, and Research). The program is designed primarily for preceptors and non-tenure-track faculty and their need to be grounded in clinical teaching, role modeling skills, the general environment of academic medicine, and the tools of research "consumerism." Some non-tenure-track faculty might possibly be drawn to this format as a way to acquire training in discrete tasks. Participants should not consider this plan adequate preparation for a tenure-track position in a university or community setting.

Two-day institutes of this type could be offered successfully at multiple sites throughout the country. Participants would select one domain each time to engage in. The entire 2-day sequence is spent in that domain, In this way, a participant would receive training in three domains per year. Participants are not expected to complete any projects or engage in studies in between the institutes. The home-base department bears very little responsibility for this experience, other than supporting the faculty member and encouraging his or her continued use of the training after the institutes are over.

Advantages

- has highly able staff or consultants in areas taught
- in-depth treatment in one topic area at a time
- provides opportunity to meet national or regional colleagues
- provides brief, uninterrupted time to address faculty skills
- provides opportunity for preceptor and non-tenure-track participants to identify with faculty role
- requires moderate expenditures

Disadvantages

- very brief training sessions
- appropriate for very limited set of competencies
- may be difficult to transfer skills learned to local setting

- no reinforcement strategies to maintain learned skills
- requires time away from practice

Implementation Map

Figure 8.5 shows how courses and other activities may be integrated and sequenced for 2-day institutes. The course numbers and titles listed on the map match those described earlier in each of the respective domains.

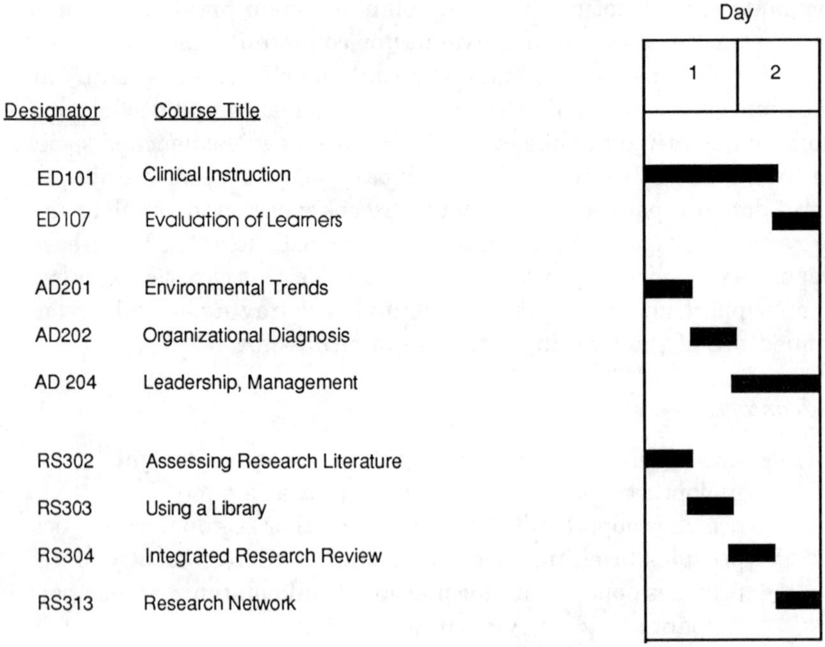

Day

		1	2

Designator	Course Title
ED101	Clinical Instruction
ED107	Evaluation of Learners
AD201	Environmental Trends
AD202	Organizational Diagnosis
AD 204	Leadership, Management
RS302	Assessing Research Literature
RS303	Using a Library
RS304	Integrated Research Review
RS313	Research Network

KEY: ■ = 1/2 Day   ■■ = 1 Day   NOTE: Participants choose one domain per institute, and institutes should be repeated 2 or 3 times a year

FIGURE 8.5 Two-day Institutes

References

Bland, C. J. , Hitchcock, M. A., Anderson, W. A., & Stritter, F. T. (1987, August). Faculty development fellowship programs in family medicine. *Journal of Medical Education, 62*(8), 632–641.

Bland, C. J., & Schmitz, C. C. (1986, January). Characteristics of the successful research and implications for faculty development. *Journal of Medical Education, 61*(1), 22–31.

CHAPTER **9**

Curriculum Evaluation

Evaluation is a critical component of any well-thought-out curriculum. The essential task of educational evaluation is to gather information to answer questions about a program—its structure and operations, activities, strengths and weaknesses, and outcomes. The purpose of answering these questions varies with the audience(s) being served and the programmatic or policy decisions to be made.

Readers will no doubt have different reasons for evaluating their faculty development programs. For example, project directors may want to better understand the strengths and weaknesses of individual strategies used in the curriculum as well as its overall format in order to revise the program before the next cycle. In contrast, teachers/presenters may be more interested in participant gains as a measure of their teaching effectiveness; such data can also indicate which methods need improvement. Faculty participants themselves will need feedback on their own progress in order to identify areas needing further development, and this requires a third instance of data-gathering and presentation. Last but not least, department chairs and their external funders will be interested in the overall merit, worth, and cost-effectiveness of the faculty development program in order to make decisions about continuing support.

Such a variety of purposes calls for a range of evaluation questions. Because the specific data and data collection strategies needed to address each of these questions will vary greatly among users, no detailed evaluation method or battery of instruments can be offered here. Rather, what we can provide are guidelines for planning and developing an evaluation. These guidelines suggest:

- an evaluation approach called the "user centered approach"
- likely questions that you, your colleagues, and funders might

ask for which systematically collected data (rather than rely-
ing on anectodal or informal evidence) is needed
- likely data to collect for the sample questions
- likely sources for these data
- likely data collection methods and study designs
- likely audiences for the evaluation information
- procedures for tailoring these suggestions to your evaluation
- general advice on planning and conducting an evaluation

Suggested Approach for Evaluation Faculty Development Programs

Before implementing an evaluation, several crucial tasks
should be accomplished. These tasks are to identify: the audience(s) (or
decision makers) who will use the evaluation information; the decisions
to be made on the basis of any information collected; the deadlines for
having evaluation data collected; and the preferred reporting format(s).
These tasks are described in Bland, Ullian, and Froberg (1984), Worthen and Sanders (1987), and Morris, Fitz-Gibbon, and Henderson (1978),
among others. Having accomplished these tasks, the evaluator works
closely with the identified decision makers to refine the specific evaluation questions and identify attainable, reliable, and valid data that
address these questions.

We suggest that readers build matrices such as the ones depicted
in Tables 9.1 and 9.2. These tables concisely summarize an evaluation
approach that is structured around questions. As can be seen, one matrix
addresses evaluation questions on the integrated curriculum level, and
the other addresses questions related to the individual domains. In the
left-hand column of each matrix, likely key evaluation questions are
listed in shortened form. (These questions are discussed in detail in the
next section, where they are listed in complete phrases.) The next
columns on the matrices are labeled *evidence* (data), *sources*, *data collection strategies*, and *audience*. Under each of these headings we have supplied examples (e.g., appropriate evidence to collect, likely sources for
those data, and possible methods for collecting data for each suggested
key question).

Key Evaluation Questions

In order to identify likely key questions, we turned to Stufflebeam's
(1971) model for evaluating educational programs, commonly called the
CIPP model. According to Stufflebeam, four major areas need to be

TABLE 9.1 Evaluation Matrix: Curriculum Level

Questions	Evidence (data)	Sources	Data Collection Strategies	Audience
1. Was the implementation plan (if adopted) appropriate for faculty and setting?	• Match between goals of plan and faculty roles and organizational mission	• Participants • Faculty • Project director • External reviewer • Needs assessment data • Mission statements • Faculty handbook	• Interview • Questionnaire • Group forum • Documents review	• Funders • Department chairs • Project directors • Faculty • Residency directors • Deans
2. Were the selected domains (if no plan was adopted) appropriate for faculty and setting?				
3. Did the curriculum (if no plan was adopted) exhibit characteristics of effective curricular design?	• Match between characteristics and written documents describing curriculum	• Project director • External reviewer	• Documents review	*
4. Was the curriculum implemented as planned? • required resources obtained? • personnel have training and experience? • courses on schedule for full time? • minimum number of participants	• Match between planned and implemented curriculum	• Program records, e.g., attendance, courses taught • Personnel vitae • Participants • Faculty • Project director • External reviews	• Interviews • Questionnaire • Document review	*
5. Was the program cost-effective	• Comparison of cost (money, resources, effort, time) estimates of own and other similar programs	• Survey of other program costs • Accounting records • Annual reports	• Survey of other programs • Interview project director, sponsors • Documents review	*

* All audiences listed for Question 1 are possible for other questions.

TABLE 9.1 Continued

Questions	Evidence (data)	Sources	Data Collection Strategies	Audience
6. Did participants achieve the goals enumerated for them in their setting?				
a. Education	• Evaluation from participants' students • Published materials • Teaching materials	• Faculty • Students • Vitae	• Interviews • Questionnaire • Materials, course records, and vitae review	*
b. Administration	• Evaluation by supervisors • Acquired leadership positions • Published materials	• Faculty • Supervisors • Vitae	• Interviews • Questionnaire • Materials, course records, and vitae review	*
c. Research	• Completed research project • Published articles • Grant proposals prepared	• Faculty • Vitae	• Interviews • Questionnaire • Materials, course records, and vitae review	*
d. Written Communication	• Completed written products—e.g., articles, books, syllabi, patient education materials, administrative documents	• Faculty • Vitae • Students • Patients • Colleagues	• Interviews • Questionnaire • Materials, course records, and vitae review	*
e. Professional Academic Skills	• Participation in University governance • Production of complete promotion packet • An established colleague network	• Participants • Department chair • P & T Committee • Colleagues • Vitae	• Interviews • Questionnaire • Materials, course records, and vitae review	*

* All audiences listed for Question 1 are possible for other questions.

TABLE 9.2 Evaluation Matrix: Domain Level

Questions	Evidence (data)	Sources	Data Collection Strategies	Audience
1. Were the competencies appropriate for the faculty and setting?	• Match between faculty responsibilities and competencies addressed	• Participants • Faculty • Project director • External reviewer • Needs assessment	• Interview • Questionnaire • Group forum • Document review	• Funders • Department chairs • Project directors • Faculty • Residency directors • Deans
2. Were the courses and formats implemented as planned? • participants attend? • teachers cover content/ competencies? • teachers perform other duties? • required materials and equipment?	• Match between planned and implemented courses			
3. How effective were the individual courses and formats?	• Course characteristics	• Participants • Program record • Program director • External reviewer/ observer	• Interview • Questionnaire • Document review • Observation	*
4. How effective were teachers/ presenters	• Teacher behaviors			

* All audiences listed for Question 1 are possible for other questions.

TABLE 9.2 Continued

Questions	Evidence (data)	Sources	Data Collection Strategies	Audience
5. Did participants' master the competencies in the domain?				
a. Education	• Participants performance on exams • Participants' students' ratings • Teacher behaviors • Teaching materials	• Participants • Students • Faculty • External reviewer/ observer • Program records	• Interview • Questionnaire • Document review • Observation	*
b. Administration	• Participants' performance on exams • Participants' diagnosis of their organization • Supervisors' evaluations	• Participants • Students • Faculty • External reviewer/ observer • Supervisor evaluations	• Interview • Questionnaire • Document review • Observation	*
c. Research	• Participants' performance on exams • Participants' research project components, e.g., literature review, data collection instruments, data analysis, articles	• Programs records • Research project reports • Faculty	• Interview • Questionnaire • Document review	*
d. Written Communication	• Participants' performance on exams • Participants' writing examples	• Program records • Faculty	• Interview • Questionnaire • Document review	*
e. Professional Academic Skills	• Participants' performance on exams • Career plans • Attitude scores	• Program records • Participants	• Interview • Questionnaire • Document review	*

* All audiences listed for question 1 are possible for other questions.

addressed when evaluating educational programs: (1) definition or structuring of the educational problem itself ("Context"); (2) conceptualization and planning of program activities ("Input"); (3) the manner in which plans were implemented ("Process"); and (4) final outcomes of learning ("Products").

Using this model as a framework, we generated potential evaluation questions at both the curriculum and domain levels. Questions under *curriculum* concern the program as a whole and the impact of each content area. Questions under *domains* concern specific features of individual domains and their courses and activities. Conceivably not every program will need to address each question, and no two programs are likely to address them to the same extent in the same manner. Still, the questions represent critical features relating to the context, input, process, and products of the faculty development curriculum.

Listed below are the key evaluation questions shown on the matrices.

Curriculum Level

1. If an implementation plan (e.g., 3- or 2-year fellowship, 12-month home off-site) was adopted, was it an appropriate plan given the needs of the faculty members involved and the goals of the particular setting?
2. If none of the implementation plans were adopted, were the domains (as selected by local planners) appropriate given the needs of faculty involved and goals of the setting?
3. If none of the implementation plans were adopted, did the curriculum (as structured by local planners) exhibit characteristics of effective curricular design (e.g., a rationale for linking courses to goals, vertical and horizontal integration of courses and other strategies, and an evaluation component)?
4. Was the resulting curriculum (program) implemented as planned? For example, (1) were the required resources (e.g., space, equipment, funding support) obtained? (2) Did the personnel (e.g., presenters, mentors, coordinators, consultants) have the required training and experience? (3) Were courses implemented on schedule for the duration planned? (4) Was the minimum numbers of participants recruited or involved?
5. Was the implemented program cost-effective?
6. Did participants achieve the goals enumerated for faculty of their type, in their setting, as identified by the local program planners?

Domain Level

1. Were the selected competencies (all or subsets) appropriate given the needs of the faculty type(s) and goals of the particular setting?
2. Were the selected courses and instructional formats implemented as planned? For example, (1) did 75% of the participants attend 75% of the time? (2) Did teachers cover as much content (i.e., address as many competencies) as planned? (3) Did teachers perform other duties (i.e., providing feedback, individual consults, referring participants to mentors) as planned? (4) Were the required materials and equipment available as expected?
3. How effective were the individual courses and other instructional formats?
4. How effective were the individual teachers/presenters and their various teaching styles?
5. Did participants master the competencies specified for the domain?

Type of Evidence (Data) to Collect.

Determining which types of evidence should be collected in order to answer the evaluation questions convincingly is an important step in evaluation. All too frequently, the type(s) of data selected are chosen simply because they are easy to collect or already exist in some relatively accessible form. Unfortunately, some of the stronger evidence of program quality can be gleaned from more difficult-to-obtain data, such as measures of observed behaviors (e.g., attendance, library requests for literature reviews), documented performances (e.g., teaching videotapes), test scores (e.g., objective tests), ratings (self or otherwise), and products (e.g., grant applications). Self-assessment and participant satisfaction data are two of the easiest to collect, but also the least valid and reliable.

The matrices include samples of evidence that would most directly answer the questions involved.

Source of Data.

The logical source for much of the data described is either the program staff or the participants. Sometimes the general literature in a particular field is also required, or a particular report or document is important. After determining the availability of desired data, the state of early records, etc., evaluators may find that they need to identify alternative forms of evidence or measures.

Collection Method and Study Design.

While the data collection strategies chosen will reflect the evaluation budget and timeline (to name just two constraints), they will also reflect the overall study design employed. Case studies, pre–post assessment (with or without a control), and experimental versus control group (post assessment only) are examples of study design. By comparison, materials review, interview, and surveys are all examples of data collection methods.

Quite a range of study designs is possible. For example, a longitudinal study comparing the number of articles produced by an experimental group with a control group could be arranged to assess a program designed to train researchers. In other areas a case study might be a preferable model. The collection methods listed as examples in the matrices demonstrate a range of strategies that could be used within a number of study designs.

Audience.

As noted earlier, likely audiences for the evaluation results are funders, program planners, presenters, and participants. Therefore, all of the possible audiences are consistently given under the heading *audience*. While such repetition would seem to make this column somewhat redundant, the inclusion (or exclusion) of a particular audience can significantly affect how questions are asked (or eliminated), how data are collected, and even who conducts the evaluation. In some cases, however, different audiences may be simultaneously served by one overall evaluation, requiring only different timelines and separate reporting formats. Lest the importance of knowing the evaluation audience be forgotten, we have retained the audience column on the matrices with its redundant examples.

Tailoring the Matrices

To use the matrices you will need to adapt them to your identified decision makers and audience(s), their questions and overall evaluation purposes, and particular features of the curriculum in your setting. If the overall evaluation purpose is summative (e.g., "Should this program continue?"), then both the curriculum- and domain-level evaluation questions (i.e., both matrices) need to be used. This is because the outcomes of domain-level strategies need to be known in order to assess curriculum-level questions. If the overall evaluation purpose is formative (e.g., "How can this program be improved?"), then the domain-level matrix may be all that is necessary. In particular, emphasis on the "process" questions (e.g., whether the courses and other strategies were implemented as planned) will be important. Thus the first step in using the components of these guidelines is to review the evaluation audiences and purposes and to select the matrices accordingly.

The second step is to adjust the questions to the curriculum as it was actually conceived or applied. If one of the implementation plans was adopted or adapted only slightly, then Question 1 on the curriculum matrix should be retained and Questions 2 and 3 dropped. If no implementation plan was adopted, or if one was selected but modified extensively, then Question 1 should be omitted and Questions 2 and 3 retained.

In addition, a careful review of the (revised) program goals and competencies needs to be made. It may be that the requisite competencies and suggested faculty development goals no longer reflect the basis of the revised curriculum format or its strategies. If evaluated under these circumstances, then the competencies and goals provided by this curriculum would provide inaccurate measures of learner achievement and, by extension, of program effectiveness. For this reason, it is very important that program planners document the goals and competencies they ultimately use.

Whatever the case, the "true" goals and competencies should be used during evaluation. If only selected subsets of the requisite competencies were adopted, then Questions 1 and 5 on the domain matrix should refer only to those subsets. If selected domains and their configuration or selected courses and other formats were radically altered, then Question 6 on 9.1, the curriculum matrix, should refer only to goals that these curricula expect to achieve.

A third step in tailoring the matrices is to generate relevant questions under Questions 4 (curriculum-level matrix) and 2 (domain matrix). Although the examples provided may be serviceable as they stand, each setting may have particular concerns in the implementation area. Additionally, some determination of "minimum requirements" needs to be made before the curriculum is implemented. By minimum requirements we mean, for example, the number of class sessions that need to be held as scheduled in order to consider the "treatment" valid; the number of participants that are required in order to make the strategy (i.e., class, seminar) "work"; the minimal sets of equipment or materials that are necessary for the program to run as planned. Obviously, if minimum requirements in such areas as budgets and participant numbers are not met, then expected outcomes must be revised.

Once the relevant questions have been written, then the appropriate data, data sources, and data collection strategies can be determined. As already outlined, the selection of these elements will be affected by the study design employed and other factors germane to each environment.

General Advice on Planning and Conducting Program Evaluation

The general approach embodied in this plan may be termed question-driven: for each evaluation question asked, specific audience(s), types of data, data sources, data collection methods, study design, analyses, and report formats are needed. A good discussion of selected study designs and data analysis strategies is found in Anderson and Ball (1980). Readers are also encouraged to review the *Standards for Evaluations of Educational Programs, Products, and Materials* (Joint Committee, 1981).

Finally, an important decision to make in conducting an evaluation is whether the evaluator should be internal or external to the organization in which the faculty development program is based. Deciding which level of evaluator to use is determined by one's resources and the audience(s) who will be interpreting, judging, and using the data. The relationship between the level of the evaluation and usefulness/credibility to various audiences is displayed in Table 9.3 (Froberg & Bland, 1981). Due to financial constraints and logistical problems, most programs will be working (perhaps exclusively) with internally integrated evaluators. And, as seen in Table 9.3, internal evaluation has high credibility and usefulness for several audiences. However, an internally segregated evaluator has more acceptable credibility with more diverse audiences. An internally segregated evaluator is one who works for the same parent organization that oversees or houses the faculty development program but is not formally a part of the program. An evaluator who is knowledgeable about faculty development generally but not directly connected with the program can provide relatively unbiased, valuable insight on the teaching skills and strategies employed, as well as on the outcomes of learning. A totally external evaluation is preferred when the primary audience is a funding agency or society and the evaluation purpose is summative only.

TABLE 9.3 The Effect of Five Evaluation Models on Desirable Qualities

Evaluation Models	Qualities							
	Freedom from Reward Structure (Independence)	Offer Fresh Perspective (Independence)	Credibility to Program Director	Credibility to Department Head	Credibility to Funding Agency, Public	Usefulness to Program Director	Usefulness to Department Head	Usefulness to Funding Agency, Public
Internal integrated	low	low	high	medium	low	high	medium	low
Internal segregated	medium	medium	medium	high	medium	medium	high	medium
External (reports to program director)	high	high	medium/high	medium/low	medium/low	medium/high	medium/low	medium/low
External (reports to department head)	high	high	low	medium/high	medium	low	medium/high	medium
External (reports to funding agency)	high	high	low	low	high	low	low	high

* This figure (adapted from Ahm 1975) is taken from Froberg, D., & Bland, C. J. (1981). *Application of internal and external evaluation models to the position and role of evaluators in a medical school department* (in-house document). Minneapolis, MN: University of Minnesota, Department of Family Practice and Community Health.

References

Anderson, S. B., Ball, S. (1980). *The profession and practice of program evaluation.* San Francisco: Jossey-Bass.

Bland, C. J., Ullian, J., & Froberg, D. (1984). User-centered evaluation. *Evaluation and the Health Professions, 7*(1), 53–63.

Froberg, D., & Bland, C. J. (1981). *Application of internal and external evaluation models to the position and role of evaluators in a medical school department* (in-house document). Minneapolis, MN: Department of Family Practice and Community Health, University of Minnesota.

Joint Committee on Standards for Educational Evaluation. (1981). *Standards for evaluations of educational programs, projects, and materials.* New York: McGraw-Hill.

Morris, L. L., Fitz-Gibbon, C. T. & Henderson, M. (1978). *Program evaluation kit.* Beverly Hills, CA: Sage.

Stufflebeam, D. L. (1971). *Educational evaluation and decision making.* Itasca, IL: Peacock.

Worthen, B. R., & Sanders, J. R. (1987). *Educational evaluation: Alternative approaches and practical guidelines.* White Plains, NY: Longman.

Guidelines for Implementing Faculty Development Programs

There is more to conducting an effective faculty development program than "just" identifying the competencies to be addressed and lining up appropriate learning strategies. To identify additional characteristics of successful programs, in-depth site visits were conducted at five successful federally funded programs (Bland & Stritter, 1988). Listed below are the critical elements of effective faculty development programs based on these visits and on extensive discussions with many other experienced faculty developers, as well as on an analysis of the literature in faculty development and our own personal experience. The critical elements are clustered into seven categories. For each category, the critical elements and discussion are presented together. When appropriate, the critical elements are discussed within the context of relevant literature.

Mission

1. A faculty development program must have a clearly stated mission or purpose that guides all decisions.
2. The faculty development program's purpose must address the needs of program faculty and individual participants.

3. the mission must be understood and supported by program faculty and individual participants.

Faculty and staff of successful programs can generally articulate the faculty development program's mission. They can explain the ways in which they contribute to it personally and how this mission serves both the larger organization and the discipline. Program directors often specify the influence their mission has on the scope, focus, and limitations of their program.

The importance of a clear mission to an effective organization is commonly accepted in organizational literature. A recent review of the past 20 years of faculty development programs in higher education (including medicine) found "clear mission" to be a critical feature of effective, enduring programs (Bland & Schmitz, 1988).

4. Project personnel should be systematic in the design and implementation of program curricula.

Directors, faculty, and participants state the importance of a clearly defined, systematic program. Most successful programs follow a systematic approach in instructional design (e.g., Gagne & Briggs, 1979).

5. Program format should be designed with specific faculty types in mind.

As emphasized throughout this book, the competencies needed by any one faculty member are largely determined by their faculty role, the priorities of their organization, and, of course, the interests and goals of individual faculty members. Faculty needs vary according to academic position and institution. Faculty development programs should address the differences between institutions, faculty roles, and individual developmental needs. The following program formats are suggested for the indicated faculty types.

5a. Preceptor
  1. Short-term formats or self-instructional materials that do not require significant time away from practice (e.g., 1- to 3-day workshops, or self-learning books, tapes, computer programs).
  2. A format in which program staff follow up sessions with several on-site visits to reinforce learning.
5b. Full-Time Non-Tenure-Track
  Programs that provide a continuous experience (e.g., year-

long with 30% time commitment) either locally or through concentrated periods (e.g., 3-day, week-long, month-long sessions) at a faculty development training site, with assignments and projects completed at home.

5.c Full-Time, University-Based, Tenure-Track
For tenure-track faculty in research-oriented universities, continuous experience (e.g., 2- to 3-year, 100% time) in a faculty development training site located in a research-oriented organization.

6. Courses should address the range of skills needed by specific participants enrolled in the program; not all faculty need all skills

Unfortunately, faculty development programs are often designed without careful assessment of the actual skills needed by the likely participants; rather, course content is determined by the expertise of available staff. In contrast, successful programs are based on the assessed needs of their participants. Participants value what they feel they will be rewarded for by their institution.

7. In addition to addressing traditional skills such as teaching, research, and administration, programs should address other faculty needs (e.g., survival skills, the academic ethic and culture, networking.)

The importance of understanding the academic culture is important. Participants should be socialized to their new role and new workplace. The literature on faculty productivity supports this. In fact, socialization to one's organization has been found to be the most important characteristic in predicting future research productivity (Bland & Schmitz, 1986).

8. Programs should have an integrated curriculum.

An integrated curriculum means that learning activities are meaningfully scheduled, either sequentially or concurrently. In this way important concepts can be reiterated across courses, in different contexts, and at more advanced levels.

To ensure an integrated program, all program faculty should be familiar with the entire program and interact frequently about their teaching. If consultants are used, they should be thoroughly oriented so their contributions complement the remainder of the curriculum.

9. Programs should emphasize both theory and practice.

Programs generally focus on the skills and abilities that participants need immediately in their work. However, programs should not focus on practice to the exclusion of theory. For example, in addition to being taught how to select a sample for a study, participants can be taught why one type of sample (e.g., random, stratified, matched) is better and what must be considered in determining appropriate sample size (e.g., power, level of statistics, population variance, and size of effect).

10. Programs should use instructional materials (printed, audio, or visual media) as a compliment to didactic sessions.

Media can greatly augment the teaching of abstract concepts, procedural sequences, and other particulars, especially for some learners. Media also supply variation and stimulation to instructional encounters. Print material has the added advantage of being transportable; faculty may get more out of a session by studying the materials at home and having them for future reference.

11. Many supervised practice opportunities, followed by specific feedback, should be part of the curriculum.

Multiple practice opportunities for newly acquired skills are characteristic of effective programs. Opportunities can be provided in such areas as teaching, curriculum development, committee leadership, organizational diagnosis, role negotiation, career planning, and research. In every instance, real or simulated practice sessions should be followed by review or observation and feedback.

12. Programs should require in-depth projects.

Supervised projects are highly effective for teaching and learning the concepts presented. Participants can better appreciate the effort required to build an educational program systematically or conduct a study as a result of successful projects. Projects can provide a tangible benefit for the program from which the participant came or to which they are going. For example, the development of a clerkship or residency curriculum with objectives, teachers' guide, syllabus, and logistics can benefit any program.

13. Programs should have mentor/advisors for participants.

Having a mentor or advisor increases the likelihood that physician faculty will receive frequent feedback and develop a constructive relationship with an academic professional. For programs with a research emphasis, the mentor is essential. Productive researchers have often found a relationship with an established researcher critical (Bland & Schmitz, 1986). While an established researcher in one's own area seems a likely choice, productive researchers in other areas can also be effective (Aran & Ben-David, 1968).

14. Full-time fellowships should have some designated time set aside for clinical practice.

The need for clinical practice during a residential fellowship is a commonly held belief among most clinical faculty and faculty development directors. The amount of time differs with type of program. Family medicine fellowships average three half-days per week; Robert Wood Johnson Foundation Fellowships suggest that clinical time take approximately 10% and NIH guidelines state that fellows should spend no more that 20% of their time in clinical practice.

15. Program staff should maintain contact with participants.

Program staff should establish and maintain contact with participants before, during, and after the program. For programs conducted both at the home site and off-site, faculty travel to and conversations with participants at their home site can be critical. Staff can identify the needs of participants and set expectations with them and their home programs. Some programs have learning contracts that each participant, home department head or residency director, and faculty development director sign together. The importance of a contact with a mentor/advisor during and after formal training has been well-established (Bland & Schmitz, 1986).

16. Program personnel should make an effort to build relationships between faculty and participants and among participants.

While learning can be exciting, it is also uncomfortable. Specifically structured opportunities for fellows and staff to get to know each other socially can be helpful. Examples of activities include picnics, dinners, role plays, and mock research conferences. These activities also facilitate networking, collaboration, and using colleagues to share ideas—all of which facilitate the work of the academician.

Personnel

17. Programs should appoint only faculty who are highly knowledgeable and committed to the program.

The "highly knowledgeable" principle can be manifest in several ways. Clinicians can teach nonmedical topics but only after they are trained in the area they are teaching. Faculty can be recruited from other academic areas or institutions. Before teaching in the program, they should attend workshops on the program, spend time in a medical clinic, read relevant medical literature, or have their sessions reviewed by the project director. Consultants can teach, particularly if the most knowledgeable instructors are desired. It is important to recruit the best experts available, but they should be trained to transfer their skills to participants.

18. Programs should consider using physicians as faculty for nonmedical topics.

Using both M.D.s and non-M.D.s as co-instructors in a faculty development program may be the best staffing solution. This approach takes advantage of experts in relevant areas (e.g., teaching, research, administration), provides medical role models, and illustrates interdisciplinary collaboration. Using both types of faculty can also trigger mutual development for the individuals on these teams. Some successful programs do not use physicians as faculty but do attempt to promote collaboration and provide role models. They work directly with fellows and judiciously use physician faculty when they illustrate particular models.

19. The project director should: commit significant time (50–100%) to faculty development; have experience as a faculty member and formally understand the functions of a faculty member; and have experience, training, and knowledge in education and faculty development. He or she should understand the clinical discipline, have leadership and staff development skills, have at least basic knowledge of all the content taught in the program, and have vision in guiding a faculty development program.

A major program—one requiring significant resources and considerable time from participants—needs a well-qualified director with formal training and experience in the areas taught and who has made a significant professional commitment to faculty development.

20. Programs should use consultants frequently and judiciously; they should always select the best in the content area.

Consultants can be used to fulfill specific functions. For example, they can be used as core staff to teach specialized topics in which program staff are not expert. Just exposing participants to role models (consultants) from other disciplines or to national leaders in the discipline or from other geographic locations can be valuable. Overuse of consultants can result in a fragmented program with inconsistent philosophies and content, however. Consultants make significant additions when they are credible, well-known, good presenters and take the time to tailor their material for the local curricula.

Participants

21. Programs should select only participants who are committed to (and have time for) improving their faculty abilities; have support from their home organizations (if involved with an off-site/on-site program); and are likely to be able to apply their skills back home.
22. For an off-site/on-site program, more then one participant should be recruited from a site—either at the same time or over time—to reinforce the application and transfer of new skills.

If the home site does not value or reward the skills learned in a faculty development program, then these skills can quickly be extinguished. Home-site colleagues and administrators sometimes fail to appreciate the time and effort it takes to develop a course or conduct research. A critical mass should be developed at each site so that new skills are reinforced and a common language is spoken.

23. Faculty development programs need to have a critical mass of participants.

A program with only one or two participants is probably ineffective for most objectives as well as not cost-effective. Therefore, a minimum of four is suggested to facilitate interaction.

Internal Relations

24. Project directors should have authority over appointing, assigning, and dismissing staff.
25. All core project staff should be involved in program design and feel ownership of it.

For faculty development programs to be effective, they must have clear leadership and a carefully selected, well-managed, trained, integrated staff who participate in programmatic decisions.

External Relations

26. The faculty development program's mission should also fit the mission of the higher organization.
27. A faculty development program must be integral to and understood and appreciated by the higher organization.
28. Programs should have real, visible, public support from the higher organization.
29. Program directors and key staff should be highly placed in the larger organization.

Again and again, these characteristics have been found to be critical to the stability and effectiveness of a faculty development program (Bland & Schmitz, 1988).

30. When using on-/off-campus formats, faculty development programs should maintain contact with and be seen as valuable to leaders in the home programs of participants.

In order for participants of on-site/off-site programs to use their newly acquired skills at home, they must be supported by the local leaders and reward structure. The faculty development program can help assure this by maintaining contact and credibility with the home program leaders.

Evaluation and Research

31. Every program should be evaluated to ascertain aspects requiring improvement.

Evaluation can be undertaken in a variety of ways, but a comprehensive effort should be made to monitor the program and ascertain weaknesses. Any aspect of a program is a potential problem and will profit from a periodic systematic review.

32. Research should be conducted on a variety of faculty development questions and issues.

Formal controlled research on the variables of faculty development is sparse compared to other areas of human behavior. Representative and accurate outcome measures should be defined and research undertaken to examine them.

References

Aran, L., & Ben-David, J. B. (1968). Socialization and career determinants of productivity of medical researchers. *Health and Social Behavior, 9*(1), 3–15.

Bland, C. J., & Schmitz, C. C. (1986). Characteristics of the successful researcher and implications for faculty development. *Journal of Medical Education, 61*(1), 22–31.

Bland, C. J., & Schmitz, C. C. (1988). Faculty vitality on review: Retrospect and prospect. *Journal of Higher Education, 59*(2), 190–224.

Bland. C. J., & Stritter, F. T. (1988). Characteristics of effective family medicine faculty development programs. *Family Medicine, 20,* 282–288.

Gagne, R. M., & Briggs, L. J. (1979). *Principles of instructional design* (2nd ed.). New York: Holt, Rinehart & Winston.

Appendix

Methods

For readers who are interested in the curriculum development methods employed in this project, the summary provided in this Appendix describes the theory, components, tasks, and research underlying our work. The text is a condensed version of the technical report that was submitted to the Division of Medicine. U.S. Department of Health and Human Services, at the end of the contract (December, 1986). For more complete summaries of the surveys and site visits, check the references for publications that have since appeared in the literature.

Curriculum Development Theory and Process

In the initial months of the contract, the authors met to discuss our methods for developing this curriculum. We elected to refine the general strategies outlined in our proposal according to the "traditional" tasks of curriculum development as defined by Tyler (1950), Taba (1962), and others. These tasks flow, theoretically, from the assessment of requisite competencies to the articulation of philosophy, to the analysis of resources and constraints, to the expression of appropriate educational goals and their rationale. The process continues with the organization of competencies into domains, the division of domains into units of study, the delineation of teaching strategies, and design of the evaluation system (see Figure A.1). Many variations of this sequence exist, but most models for developing curriculum and instruction identify steps similar to those outlined by Tyler.

1. Sources for Objectives (Compentencies)

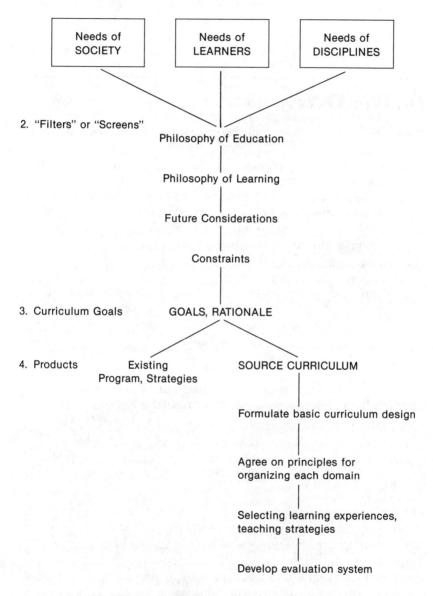

FIGURE A.1 Curriculum development model.

Adapted from Ralph Tyler (1950). *Basic principles of curriculum and instruction.*
Chicago: University of Chicago Press.

Tyler's curriculum development model served us in several ways. First, it helped us identify the appropriate sources (i.e., constituents and bodies of literature) for identifying the requisite competencies. Tyler would have used the word "objectives" rather than "competencies," but the underlying strategy of tapping a constellation of sources for educational needs in the same. Tyler's three sources for determining school curriculum objectives are the society (i.e., school community), the learners (i.e., elementary/secondary students), and the disciplines (i.e., subject matter or content areas such as English, history, etc.). To determine the appropriate objectives in Tyler's model, the needs of each of these sources are gathered, weighed, and translated into behaviorally stated objectives of learning. In our terminology, these objectives represent skills (competencies) that faculty members need to master.

For our purposes, we operationalized Tyler's sources as follows: (1) *Society* signifies the family medicine department and affiliated university or hospital program. This group or "source" has several needs and priorities concerning faculty development. Generally, these needs concern the ability of faculty members to fulfill certain roles, to subscribe to professional values or codes of behavior, and to perform required tasks within the institution. (2) *Learners* translates to current, past, and future faculty development participants. These physician participants need to master a host of nonclinical skills in addition to clinical skills in order to succeed as faculty members in their setting. (3) *Discipline* comprises the necessary knowledge and skills in the relevant content domains of the faculty development curriculum. To illustrate the needs of the discipline, consider the possible answers to the questions: "In order to teach, or to conduct research (etc.) well, what do faculty participants need to learn?" "What concepts and skills does mastery in written communication imply?" Tyler's model suggests that by combining input from the society, the learners, and the discipline, appropriate requisite faculty competencies can be determined.

Project staff also adopted what we believed to be Tyler's implied definition of the term "curriculum." In our approach to the contract, we understood "curriculum" to denote both *content* ("Which skills, concepts, subjects should be taught?") and *process* ("How should these skills, etc., be taught to these learners given these constraints and goals?"). This definition also fits the terms of the contract, which indicated that both contents (e.g., requisite competencies) and process (e.g., learning experiences and strategies) should be addressed. We therefore prepared documents that contain components that the curriculum literature suggests should be present in materials designed to address both content and process. These components are listed below. They were guided by Tyler (1950) and Taba (1962), Gall (1984), and others.

Components of Curricular Products

1. *Philosophy.* The purpose and nature of faculty development; the process and context of learning faculty skills.
2. *Goals.* Faculty development aims for different types of faculty.
3. *Content Domains.* Content areas that faculty developers need to address: Education, Administration, Research, Written Communication, Professional Academic Skills.
4. *Requisite Competencies.* Specific skills in each area that faculty need to learn.
5. *Learning Formats and Activities.* Developed sequences of courses, experiences, and strategies.
6. *Materials.* References to existing texts and course materials; annotated bibliography.
7. *Implementation.* Plans for integrating courses across domains into programs for different types of faculty.
8. *Evaluation.* Evaluation design, questions, and guidelines for assessing learners' progress and program effectiveness.

Curriculum Development Tasks

Over the course of two-and-one-half years we employed several methods to produce these components, including literature reviews, consensus meetings with key representatives, collaboration between content experts, surveys, collection of existing materials, site visits, and a "paper pilot" (external review by experts). These methods were applied to achieve the process steps indicated in Tyler's model.

First, we set about the task of preparing requisite competencies by generating data from our three identified sources—the department chairs and program directors in family medicine ("society"), the faculty participating in faculty development programs ("learners"), and the literature and experts in related fields and subjects ("discipline"). To obtain these data, we searched the literature in five content domains, developed surveys, and met with our physician liaisons, department and faculty members, and committee members.

Second, we again drew upon the literature to develop a philosophy of family medicine faculty development. Third, we set about the tasks of defining relevant faculty development goals by surveying relevant groups (department chairs, residency directors, and faculty alumni). After collecting existing faculty development materials from existing programs and site-visiting five program locations, we finally drafted curricular materials.

These steps are illustrated in Figure A.2 and further explained in the text that follows. Generally speaking, all the activities in the first 18 months of the contract involved data gathering and assessment. Activities devoted to curriculum design, testing, and documentation dominated the last 12 months of the project.

Key to Figure A.2—Explanation of Curriculum Development Tasks

1. Literature review by content experts in education, administration, research, written communication, and professional academic skills; faculty development; and other areas to identify appropriate domains and their requisite skills (Fall 1984 through Spring 1985). (Source: *Discipline*)

2. A request for all existing faculty development materials from family medicine project directors funded by Department of Health and Human Services, Robert Wood Johnson Foundation, Kellogg Foundation and other sources (Fall 1984). (Source: *Discipline and Society*)

3. First draft of requisite competencies based on the literature (Winter through Spring 1985). (Source: *Discipline and Society*)

4. Review and critique of competencies by physician liaisons (Spring 1985). (Source: *Society*)

5. Consensus meetings and informal survey of department chairs and faculty members serving on our advisory committee to gather their views on the requisite competencies (May 1985). (Source: *Society*)

6. Survey study of graduates of family medicine faculty development fellowship programs to determine how essential requisite competencies are for success in community- and university-based programs, and the effectiveness of particular training formats and strategies (Summer 1985). (This study was co-funded by the Robert Wood Johnson Foundation and the Division of Medicine, Department of Health and Human Services, through HRSA #84 592(p). It was conducted by the Society of Teachers of Family Medicine Task Force on Faculty Development, Carole Bland, Chair.) The results of this study were later published (Bland, Hitchcock, Anderson, & Stritter, 1987; Hitchcock, Anderson, Stritter & Bland, 1988). (Source: *Learners*)

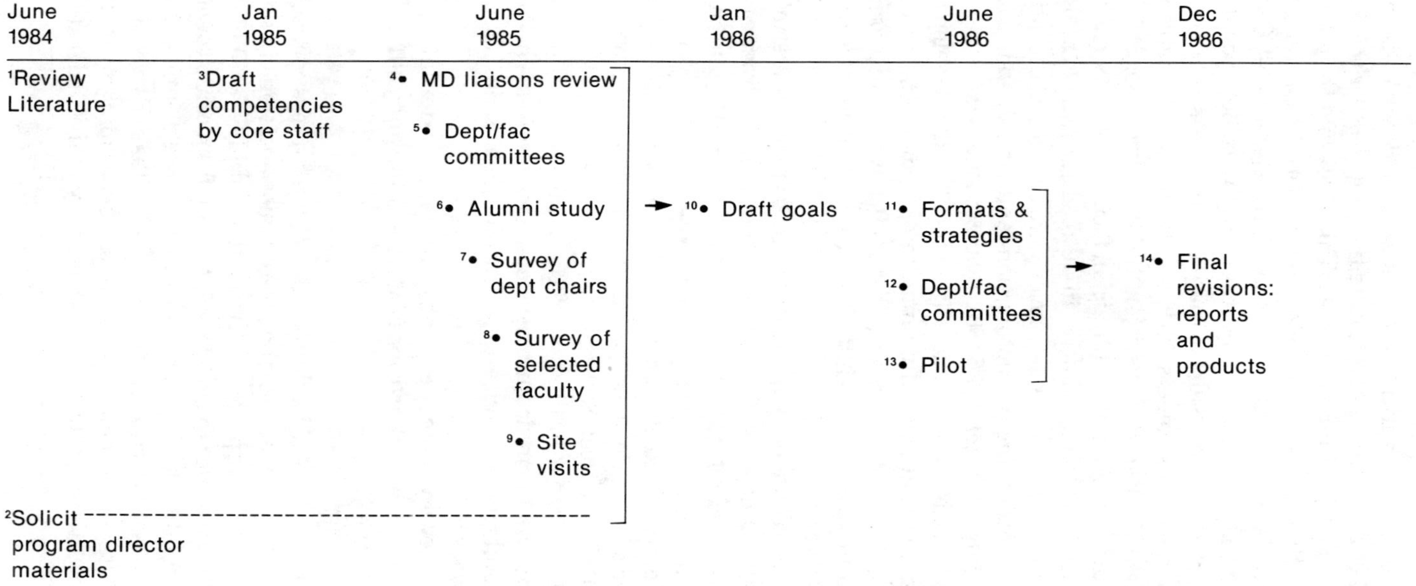

FIGURE A.2 Key events: contract in family medicine faculty development.

7. Survey of department chairs and residency directors to fur-
    ther differentiate appropriate training goals for the three types
    of faculty (Winter 1985–86). (This study and the one described
    in #8, were funded by and conducted at the University of Min-
    nesota and the University of North Carolina at Chapel Hill
    by the contract's project staff. They were not specified by the
    contract.) The results of these studies were summarized in two
    in-house documents (Stritter, Bland, & Youngblood, 1986;
    Schultz, Bland, & Stritter, 1986). (Source: *Society*)

8. Survey of exemplary physician faculty in family medicine and
    other clinical specialties in 50 medical schools to determine
    which requisite competencies were considered essential by the
    top-performing preceptors, non-tenure-track and tenure-track
    faculty (Winter 1985–86). (Source: *Learners*)

9. Site visits to five federally funded faculty development pro-
    grams to further illuminate project directors' and program
    leaders' views on training needs, effective training formats, and
    future priorities (Winter 1985 through Spring 1986). (Source:
    Society)

10 & 11. Draft of goals, curriculum formats, and strategies by
    content experts after reviewing previous data from various sur-
    veys and incorporating the literature review and input from
    other sources (Spring 1986). (Source: *All*)

12. Review of the goals, curricular formats, and strategies by phy-
    sician liaisons and department and faculty committees (Spring
    1986). (Source: *Society*)

13. An external evaluation of the complete curriculum by four
    experts in curriculum development, family medicine, faculty
    development, and evaluation (Summer 1986). (Source: *Dis-
    cipline*)

14. Review by content experts (core staff) of external evaluations,
    leading to final revisions for reports and and deliverables (Fall
    1986).

As the key to Figure A.2 explains, three of the surveys conducted were
not specified by the contract; they were major additions to the methodology outlined in our proposal. Two of these studies were undertaken
by project staff in order to gather information from constituent sources
other than the literature, our committee members, and consultants.
The third was undertaken by the STFM Task Force on Faculty
Development for a number of purposes. These surveys are described
briefly below, along with the site visit study of five federally funded
programs.

1. *Study of Graduates of Family Medicine Faculty Development Fellowship Programs*

This study was conducted by the STFM Task Force on Faculty Development from September 1984 to March 1986 (Bland, Hitchcock, Anderson, & Stritter, 1986, 1987). Cofunded by the Robert Wood Johnson Foundation (RWJ) and the Division of Medicine of the Department of Health and Human Services (HHS), the intent of this project was to study the graduates of both RWJ and HHS fellowship training programs. By 1984, several hundred alumni had participated in 3-, 6-, 9-, and 12-month and 2-year fellowships, and funders wished to know more about the current roles of these graduates and by implication the impact of their training programs.

Of the seven major study questions addressed in a survey to 329 graduates, several were of particular importance to this curriculum. The investigators (Bland, Hitchcock, Anderson, & Stritter) asked alumni to review a list of requisite faculty skills (competencies) and to rate how essential these skills were for success for faculty in their roles and institutional setting. Alumni were also asked how much emphasis was placed on these same skills during their fellowship programs. These competencies were grouped into five areas. Forty-one in total, they were condensed versions of the original list of 226 competencies derived from the literature by the content experts on this project.

This survey yielded valuable information about the competencies that graduates valued and about the perceived amount of emphasis these skills received in responding alumni's past fellowship programs. Through this survey, therefore, we were able to fulfill our objective of gathering data on learners' needs. This survey also produced data on the characteristics of successful faculty development programs. Clearly, certain program features (such as format and length) were essential for achieving particular development goals. This information was useful to us as we constructed the implementation plans and domain-level curricula.

2. *Survey of Department Chair and Residency Directors on Selected Faculty Types and Subsequent Faculty Development Goals*

This study was conducted by core staff (Schmitz, Bland, & Stritter, 1986) in November/December 1985 with the support of the Universities of Minnesota and North Carolina at Chapel Hill. Its purpose was to better understand how faculty members' roles were defined in community and university settings and to identify which faculty development goals were considered essential for various faculty members by their department or program leaders. We felt that in order for model curricula to be successful, faculty development competencies and strategies should be linked to the target audiences and institutional goals in an appropriate fashion.

We therefore designed a questionnaire in two parts and distributed it to all family medicine department chairs (N=111) and residency directors (N=383) in the United States. The survey's first part offered descriptions of three faculty types (tenure-track, non-tenure-track, and preceptor) and asked respondents to identify how well these descriptions matched faculty on their staff in those positions and to comment on the discrepancies. We then presented a list of 25 possible goals of faculty development. Respondents rated how essential these goals were for each faculty type in their setting.

By comparing the responses of department chairs (54%) with residency directors (44%), we were able to isolate differences in priorities between the two settings. Their responses also informed us of the differences in expectations for faculty in different roles. This survey was very instrumental for understanding the range of faculty types and their distribution in university and community settings. It therefore fulfilled our objective of querying "society" members about important faculty needs and valued developmental goals.

3. *Survey of Exemplary Medical Faculty Identified by Fifty Offices of Medical Education*

This study was also conducted by core staff (Stritter, Bland & Young-blood, 1986) during the fall of 1985 with the support of their two universities. Its purpose was to directly test the importance of requisite competencies (N=211) as derived by literature review and revised after meetings with our advisory committees. Once again we wanted to understand how essential these faculty skills were for success for different types of faculty in university and community settings. In this survey, however, we asked not only family medicine physician faculty but also faculty in six other primary care medical specialties (including pediatrics, internal medicine, and obstetrics and gynecology) to review and rate the competencies. Further, we looked only at a selected group of exemplary faculty. These individuals were recommended to us by 50 offices of medical education in the U.S. and primary care department chairs and residency directors. The following lists how many completed questionnaires were returned (and how many sent) for each type of faculty member: non-family medicine tenured or tenure track, 56 (of 73); family medicine tenured or tenure track, 74 (of 108); family practice non-tenure track, 91 (of 120); and preceptors, 55 (of 101).

Our motivation for surveying top-performing faculty is consistent with the literature in instructional systems, which suggests that "master performers" can be used as a source for educational objectives. The theory is that the most accomplished individuals will be able to identify which skills are critical for success; they will be able to tell you what is important to teach others.

Also it seemed important to know which competencies were considered important by the larger "society" in which academic physician faculty are a part. Physician faculty, after all, are not being developed to meet only local or internal expectations, but also to meet external requirements of the medical school and university. These constituents, as represented by exemplary faculty outside of family medicine, needed to be queried.

4. *Final Report on Federal Training (Study of Five Federally Funded Faculty Development Programs in Family Medicine)*

In order to ascertain the impact of federal guidelines on faculty development program formats and content, to identify characteristics of successful programs, and to gather recommendations for future programs, project staff visited five programs: the Faculty Development Center sponsored by the McLennan County Medical Education and Research Foundation in Waco, Texas, and programs at the University of North Carolina, Michigan State University, University of Miami, and Duke University (Bland & Stritter, 1986a, 1988). Visits began during the winter of 1985–86 and continued through the summer of 1986. The site visit consisted of a daylong series of interviews with project directors and staff, faculty participants, and department chair or supervisor and a review of relevant materials.

Study findings consisted of recommendations concerning future funding guidelines and guidelines for effective faculty development programs. These later guidelines affected the implementation of programs—and therefore the implementation sections of this curriculum—most heavily.

A final note on the execution of tasks outlined in Figure A.2: although we hoped to incorporate existing teaching materials in family medicine faculty development, we were unable to do so for several reasons. We contacted 39 project directors in the fall of 1984 and asked to share references to articles, existing reports, and whatever teaching materials they used in their programs. The response rate on our request for basic contact information was high ($N = 30$, or 76%), but the quantity of teaching materials actually submitted was low. Few project directors sent materials other than brochures, an occasional evaluation report, or a grant application. We learned that for many project directors teaching materials are proprietary. Other project directors considered them useful in-house but unsuitable for dissemination because of their rough form. For these reasons, we incorporated few existing materials into the curriculum (other than our own), although several references appear in various domains.

In summary, the contract's modus operandi was to implement tasks suggested by the curriculum development literature as outlined by Tyler and specified in the key steps of the contract. These tasks included literature review, consensus meetings with advisory committees, the use of three surveys, five site visits, collaboration among content experts, and an external evaluation.

Summary of Findings From Data-Gathering Tasks

As previously mentioned, the purpose of conducting literature reviews, surveys, consensus meetings, site visits, and other tasks was to provide a base of information on which to build a model curriculum. Primary findings from the events just outlined fall into three categories, as outlined below:

1. *Faculty abilities in academic medicine.* Findings relating to the generic nature of requisite faculty competencies; the relevance of academic medical competencies to family medicine and other primary care physicians
2. *Faculty development needs in family medicine.* Findings relating to the range of faculty roles and positions in academic family medicine and the relevance of requisite competencies to each faculty role.
3. *Faculty development program models.* Findings relating to the suitability and range of program models for the range of faculty needs.

Each of these topics will be discussed in the sections that follow.

Faculty Abilities in Academic Medicine

Our search for requisite faculty abilities began with a look at the family medicine literature but quickly led to the broader disciplines of education, organizational development, research methods, English rhetoric, professional socialization, and beyond. The search for competencies, in other words, did not begin by isolating abilities known to be important to family medicine faculty only, but with abilities believed to be important for all physician faculty, or to faculty members in higher education generally. This approach generated a list that was initially "discipline-free" to an extraordinary extent. The preliminary draft of competencies based on the literature was quite generic. Then, through the subsequent methods of further review, consensus meetings, collaboration, surveys, and several revisions, the competencies were tailored to more specific needs of preceptors, non-tenure-track, and tenure-track faculty in primary care.

We believe the final list accurately reflects the range of skill needs required by academic medical faculty *as a group*. Probably no single faculty member could be expected to master all the skills, although there is considerable evidence that the full-time, tenure-track faculty member has greatest need for the highest number of them. But collectively, physician faculty as a group need to master these skills to perform their collective roles well. This master list was confirmed by department and faculty advisors and the four external reviewers, each of whom felt the content was valid for academic medicine. Each of these individuals expressed preferences in terms of language and level of detail and cited alternate sources of literature, but none suggested that any segments of the final list be dropped, nor did they suggest that any areas be added.

The list of competencies remains, therefore, a fairly generic creature—logically so, perhaps, for the skills of presenting a lecture, evaluating a student, conducting a committee meeting, writing a report, and so forth do not change radically (if at all) with the specialty or discipline. The content being taught, evaluated, or discussed changes, and content can "color" or highlight the skills being used in distinctive ways. Still, the requisite nonclinical competencies represent process skills germane to many faculty members, both within and outside the medical school.

Results from the Survey of Exemplary Faculty further reveal how generic the list of competencies is. Our instrument used a 4-point scale in which a 2 designated "useful but not required," a 3 indicated "highly desirable but not essential," and a 4 meant "essential." As Table A.1 shows, the competencies were rated fairly highly by all respondents across specialties with the exception of preceptors. The mean scores for competencies in research (3.33), professional academic skills (3.17), written communication (3.20), and teaching (3.08) all approached the "essential" range for non-family-medicine respon-

TABLE A.1 Mean Scores of Essentialness by Domain According to Exemplary Faculty in Family Medicine and Other Specialties

Domains	Non-family* Medicine	Family Medicine Preceptors	Family Medicine Non-tenure-track	Family Medicine Tenure-track
Research	3.33 (1)	2.79 (5)	2.83 (5)	3.17 (4,5)
Teaching	3.08 (4)	3.17 (1)	3.29 (1)	3.23 (2)
Administration	2.70 (5)	2.99 (2)	3.11 (2)	3.17 (4,5)
Written communication	3.20 (2)	2.98 (3)	3.10 (3)	3.20 (3)
Professional academic skills	3.17 (3)	2.84 (4)	3.08 (4)	3.26 (1)
Total mean	3.06	2.84	3.04	3.17

* All non-family-medicine respondents were in tenure-track positions or tenured.

dents. Ratings for competencies by family medicine tenure-track faculty were even higher; they surpassed the 3.0 mark in all five domains, although the rank order was different when compared to that of non-family practice faculty. (For example, professional academic competencies were considered most essential by family practice faculty in tenure-track positions, followed by teaching, writing, and administration and research. The priorities of other faculty outside of family medicine were in research writing, and professional academic skills; teaching was listed fourth.)

Non-tenure-track faculty also rated the competencies in four of the five domains highly (3.0 or above). Their mean ratings were slightly below those of tenure-track faculty in administration, written communication, and professional academic skills. Their ratings of teaching skills were actually higher—and the highest of any faculty group for this domain. In contrast, research was the only domain to score below 3.0. Only preceptors rated research lower than did non-tenure-track family medicine faculty.

We especially noted the differences between family medicine and non-family-medicine faculty in their ratings of research competencies. Family practice faculty considered teaching skills more essential than research skills, and rated research skills lower than did their non-family-medicine counterparts. This discrepancy in priority between teaching and research is slight for tenure-track faculty, more noticeable for non-tenure-track faculty.

The conclusions we drew from this survey were several. First, the list of competencies itself describes rather generic faculty abilities that are considered highly desirable (if not essential) by faculty in academic medicine. Second, we concluded that the ratings of tenure-track faculty in family medicine are similar to those of non-family-medicine faculty in terms of importance, but not priority. The difference between the ranks is small, but possibly important. Third, we noted that the competencies as a whole were deemed less important by preceptors. Fourth, we took special note of the high rating of professional academic skills by tenure-track faculty in family medicine. This priority may indicate how difficult the transition to academe has been for this group.

In summary, we learned from the literature review and survey of exemplary faculty that nonclinical faculty competencies are generalizable across medical specialties within primary care. Their basis in higher education literature, organizational development, and other areas suggests they are relevant to other health professionals as well.

Faculty Development Needs in Family Medicine

To understand further how the requisite competencies apply to preceptors, non-tenure-track, and tenure-track faculty, we examined the interaction between faculty role (as represented by academic position) and institutional setting. One of the initial objectives of the contract was to explicate the differences between faculty development needs in university and community settings and to accommodate these differences in our curricula. Although distinctions between settings certainly do exist, we found that faculty's academic position was the dominant predictor of development needs.

Therefore, the critical question was: "Which competencies are requisite for which type of faculty and to what degree?" The answer depended on the manner in which faculty roles and priorities were defined in each setting. If faculty were expected to secure research funding and design and manage studies, for example, fairly obvious skills in research design and analysis were considered essential. In contrast, if faculty were expected to merely read and apply ("consume") research but not conduct it, a more limited set of skills was generally recommended.

We gained this understanding of the range of faculty roles from the Survey of Department Heads and Residency Directors, administered to all family practice program directors and department chairs in December 1985. First, we learned that the definition we provided (see Chaper 1) for tenure-track, non-tenure-track, and preceptor faculty met with widespread agreement. (These descriptions highlight what have been commonly accepted role differences, with emphasis leaning either toward research or toward teaching and patient care.) Ninety percent of the department chairs agree that our description of non-tenured-track faculty matched faculty of the category in their setting; agreement reached 94% for the tenure-track description, and 97% for the preceptor description. Agreement from residency directors was also impressively high for the preceptor and non-tenure-track description (99% and 94% respectively). The percentage of agreement dropped to 76% for tenure-track faculty descriptions, but this figure can still be considered substantial.

We also found that different settings employed a somewhat different mix of faculty types. While virtually all respondents reported having preceptors on their staff (department chair = 100%, residency directors = 93%), department chairs were twice as likely to employ tenure-track faculty as residency directors. Eighty-five percent of the responding departments reported tenure-track faculty, compared to 30% of the residencies. More residency directors employed non-tenure-track faculty than did department chairs (89% to75%, respectively).

This means that more than two thirds of all tenure-track faculty are in university settings. In contrast, preceptors are employed by almost every department or program in the country, be they university- or community-based. Non-tenure-track faculty positions occur in roughly three quarters of both settings.

The demographics of the two primary settings were also interesting to compare. Most departments employed between 1 and 50 preceptors, 1 to 10 non-tenure-track faculty, and 1 to 10 tenure-track faculty. In comparison, the majority of residency programs had between 1 and 25 preceptors, 1 to 5 non-tenure-track faculty, and 1 to 5 tenure-track faculty. Therefore, although there were fewer departments than residency programs, they tended to have larger faculty bodies in every category (tenure-track, non-tenure-track, and preceptor).

An illustration of how essential the requisite competencies were considered by young faculty in these different academic positions was obtained in the Study of Graduates of Family Medicine Faculty Development Programs. In the summer of 1985, graduates of RWJ and HHW fellowship programs—then in faculty positions—rated the essentialness of 41 requisite competencies. (These were a matched subset of a complete list of competencies used in the survey of exemplary faculty.) Their responses were analyzed according to the faculty positions of full-time tenure-track, full-time non-tenure-track, and part-time (volunteer or paid preceptor). Results showed that tenure-track faculty rated competencies in each of the five domains (mean total) more essential than either non-tenure-track or preceptor faculty (see Table A.2).

Moreover, differences in the rank order of the domains appeared between tenure-track and non-tenure-track faculty. In fact, the responses from tenure-track and non-tenure-track faculty mirrored each other; one list of priorities was almost the inverse of the other. For the tenure-track faculty member, research, written communication, and professional academic skills were most important (in that order), with administration and teaching skills considered least essential (although still highly desirable). For non-tenure-track faculty, only professional academic skills were considered highly desirable; teaching, administration, written communication, and research followed in descending order.

Table A.3 compares the ratings of alumni with exemplary faculty in family medicine and other medical specialties.In looking at their mean totals (see Table A.3), we found that fellowship alumni currently in tenure-track faculty positions rated the competencies highest of any faculty group, followed by exemplary family medicine faculty (tenure-track) and faculty in other specialties. Non-tenure-track faculty in family medicine rated the competencies lowest.

TABLE A.2 Mean Scores of Essentialness by Domain According to Family Medicine Fellowship Alumni

Domains	Full-time Tenure-track	Full-time Non-tenure-track	Part-time Preceptor or Volunteer
Teaching	3.06 (5)	2.99 (2)	2.82 (2)
Administration	3.13 (4)	2.94 (3)	2.28 (5)
Research	3.46 (1)	2.79 (5)	2.47 (4)
Written communication	3.30 (2)	2.91 (4)	2.57 (3)
Professional academic skills	3.25 (3)	3.10 (1)	2.88 (1)
Total mean	3.24	2.94	2.60

* Scale: 0 = Can't judge; 1 = Unessential; 2 = Useful but not required;
  3 = Highly desirable but not essential; 4 = Essential for success

TABLE A.3 Rank Order of Mean Scores of Essentialness of Skills According to Family Medicine Fellowship Alumni and Exemplary Faculty in Family Medicine and Other Specialties

Rank Order	Exemplary* Non-family Medicine	Fellowship Alumni Tenure-track	Exemplary Family Medicine Tenure-track	Fellowship Alumni Non-tenure-track
1	Research (3.33)	Research (3.46)	P.A.S.** (3.26)	P.A.S. (3.10)
2	P.A.S. (3.17)	P.A.S. (3.25)	Teach (3.23)	Teach (2.99)
3	Writing (3.20)	Writing (3.30)	Admin (3.17)	Admin (2.94)
4	Teach (3.08)	Admin. (3.13)	Research (3.17)	Writing (2.91)
5	Admin. (2.70)	Teach (3.06)	Writing (3.20)	Research (2.79)
Mean total	3.06	3.24	3.17	2.94

* All non-family medicine respondents were tenured or in tenure-track positions.
** P.A.S. refers to Professional Academic Skills.

When the responses to individual domains were examined and rank-ordered, we found interesting similarities among the faculty groups. Tenure-track alumni's priorities most resembled those of non-family-medicine exemplary faculty; each listed research competencies as most essential, and teaching and administration as least essential. Again, an inverse priority was seen in the responses of the other faculty groups. Exemplary family medicine (tenure-track) faculty and alumni now in non-tenure-track positions felt that professional academic skills and teaching were most relevant for their tasks; research and written communication were least relevant. Our primary conclusion from Tables A.1–A.3 is that more competencies are considered essential for tenure-track and non-tenure-track positions than for preceptors.

Another illustration of how faculty needs were separated by academic position was seen in the Survey of Department Heads and Residency Directors. In this survey, department chairs and residency directors rated goals of development rather than competencies. They addressed the question: "How essential is it that faculty development programs enable faculty to" accomplish 25 possible goals for faculty in their own setting. Respondents rated each goal separately for the tenure-track, non-tenure-track, and preceptor faculty on their staff.

For this survey, a scale identical to the one used in the Survey of Exemplary Faculty was used. The mean responses of department chairs were found for each goal. Those are listed under UB (university-based) in Table A.3 which fell at or above the midpoint between the top two options on the scale. Similarly, the mean responses of residency directors were found for each goal, and the essential items are X'd under CB (community-based) in Table A.4.

TABLE A.4 Essential Faculty Development Goals in Community and University Settings According to Department Chairs and Residency Directors

[N = 61(UB), 170(CB)]*

"How essential is it that faculty development programs enable faculty to . . ."	Precept UB	CB	Non-tenure-track UB	CB	Tenure-track UB	CB
1. Be familiar with the educational ("home-base") program and the specific course/rotation their students take			X	X	X	
2. Understand the scope and sequence of the undergraduate and graduate curriculum and the place of their content or teaching within the curriculum			X		X	
3. Keep current in clinical skills and knowledge	X	X	X	X	X	X
4. Access medical and educational literature relevant to their areas of practice and need			X	X	X	X
5. Continuously build in-depth knowledge in a research content area (e.g., "compliance") and access other relevant areas of medical and educational literature					X	
6. Understand fundamental principles and procedures of research (i.e., research design and data collection)					X	X
7. Obtain research grants					X	
8. Obtain training grants					X	
9. Design and implement research studies					X	

TABLE A.4 *Continued*

10. Communicate results of research by publishing, giving presentations					X	X
11. Understand the nature and tasks of effective mentoring/role modeling	X	X	X	X	X	X
12. Teach individuals and small groups in clinical settings	X	X	X	X	X	X
13. Design educational programs, courses, units of instruction					X	
14. Deliver instruction through a broad variety of formats, including lecture, small and large group discussions, tutoring, individualized learning					X	X
15. Understand the principles of teaching and of learning in depth					X	
16. Articulate to students a clinical reasoning process and management style	X	X	X	X	X	X
17. Complete student evaluations, course or program assessment forms, and procedures	X		X	X	X	X
18. Develop assessment instruments to evaluate students, courses, programs						
19. Administer residency, undergraduate, and predoctoral programs						
20. Supervise clinic operations						
21. Work productively in committees and groups, as leaders or participants				X	X	X
22. Communicate effectively in administrative writing, student and patient materials					X	X
23. Discuss questions of medical ethics and the professional values of the practitioner				X		
24. Manage their professional and personal growth			X	X	X	X
25. Serve the discipline and profession by establishing and maintaining networks, serving in organizations, consulting, etc.					X	

* UB = University-based (Department chair responses)
   CB = Community-based (Residency Director responses)

Five of the six possible faculty groups found in Table A.4 can be clustered into one of three categories, based on the responses of department chairs and residency directors and their development priorities. These groups are (1) preceptors (either university- or community-based), (2) non-tenure-track faculty (either setting), and (3) university-based, tenure-track faculty. Both the number and type of goals considered essential for these groups were different (see Table A.5). For example, both sets of respondents considered only 4 of the 25 development goals essential for preceptors. Non-tenure-track faculty required 9 to 11 goals (depending on the setting), whereas university=based tenure-track faculty required 20 goals. The emphasis for non-tenure-track faculty was on teaching goals. The tenure-track role in universities emphasized research but covered virtually every area.

The only faculty type that does not fit readily into one of the above categories is the community-based tenure-track faculty members, a relatively rare creature employed in approximately 30% of the community settings (see Table A.5). This faculty member apparently has distinct needs and is therefore unlike both university-based tenure-track and community-based non-tenure-track faculty. According to their program leaders, these faculty require more emphasis on research and a bit less on teaching than their community colleagues, but overall much less development than their university counterparts.

In summary, our respondents to the three surveys represented different constituent sources (i.e., learners, society). All were able to differentiate the several faculty roles and identify similar priorities for skill development. As such, there is considerable empirical support for linking training goals and competencies to specific types of faculty as defined by their role expectations in the setting. The purpose for doing so, however, is not to force prescribed goals onto particular faculty members or to discriminate against certain faculty by withholding instruction in areas they wish to pursue. Rather, understanding faculty types and their needs ensures that we design programs with proper scope and emphasis for the majority of faculty who do fit well into one category or another.

Readers should also note that the Survey of Department Heads and Residency Directors influenced this project's goals, but that the two lists of goals are not identical. Final goals for the curricula was derived by content experts after reviewing all the surveys and literature review findings and preparing their competencies. But again, this final list of goals should not be interpreted as a mandate (e.g., that non-tenure-track faculty do not need to write well or conduct research). In fact, it is critical that departments assess their own mission and needs and tailor these faculty development goals.

TABLE A.5 Comparison Between Three Faculty Types on Number
of Essential Faculty Development Goals

| Preceptors | | Non-tenure-track | | Tenure-track | |
UB*	CB	UB	CB	UB	CB
5	4	9	11	21	11

* UB = university-based; CB = community-based.

Faculty Development Program Models

Our investigation of faculty development curricula and program
models began with a look at existing faculty development programs.
We reviewed three sources of data concerning existing programs: (1)
the collection of project directors' materials gathered for this contract,
(2) the study of federally funded programs by Bland, Dalgaard, Moo-
Dodge, and Froberg (1985), and (3) the site visit data (Final Report
on Federal Training) by Bland and Stritter (1986a, 1988). A brief summary of our findings is provided below.

Project Director Materials
Between August 1 and September 15, 1984, we solicited materials
from 39 project directors funded by the federal government and the
Robert Wood Johnson and Kellogg Foundations. Thirty project directors responded to our request for updated contact information; 15 sent
a variety of materials that we scrutinized for goals, instructional formats, targeted faculty audiences, and evaluation strategies.

What we found can best be described as a potpourri of programs,
program goals, and instructional formats Five respondents said their
programs covered "all" faculty types. Three responding programs targeted community preceptors; four programs were geared toward the
"new, full-time academically oriented" participants. Four others were
suitable for existing university-based faculty. Two programs were
aimed at residents; one specified "anyone who teaches," but specifically family practice program directors or assistant directors.

The 15 respondents cited goals or objectives in 13 content areas:
education ($N=10$), research ($N=7$), administration ($N=5$), computers
($N=3$), professional development ($N=3$), and evaluation ($N=3$). Goals
in professional communication (oral or written) and clinical care were
stated by two programs. Health care delivery systems, recruitment
of new faculty, family medicine content, interpersonal relationships,
and medical ethics were stated by one program each.

Instructional formats also ran the gamut from supervised patient care to consultation, individualized learning (materials or computers), 1- or 2-day workshops, and 5- or 6-week programs. The 1-year fellowship (N=5) and the seminar series of six to nine sessions (N=6) were the two most prevalent strategies in this sample. One-week institutes (N=1) were the least frequent.

In terms of an evaluation component, again an array of strategies was cited in the materials, although only a handful of programs reported any systematic evaluation system. The following strategies were cited by several programs: student evaluations of faculty, objective tests, attendance counts, participant survey, staff report, peer review, rating of audiotape or videotape, interviews, and external program evaluation.

Study of Federally Funded Faculty Development
The data summarized above were echoed with greater clarity by a broader survey of faculty development programs funded between 1978 and 1981 in family medicine. The authors of this study found that project participants were of three types: paid faculty (full- or part-time), volunteers, and fellows. The biggest group addressed was the full- or part-time, paid faculty member; the next largest was the volunteer group. The smallest participant group was composed of fellows (Bland, Dalgaard, Moo-Dodge, and Froberg (1985).

All projects cited one common goal: "improving faculty teaching skills." Additional goals (in descending order of frequency) were to improve faculty research skills (83%), develop curriculum (75%), increase full-time faculty (61%), improve faculty skills in the clinical area (61%), and improve faculty skills in administration (56%).

A variety of formats and teaching strategies were used. Interestingly enough, nearly all major formats were used to address each goal, even across projects. The most common instructional strategy cited was 1-day workshops. The 2-day workshop was the next most prevalent form of development, followed by 6-week seminars, episodic consultation, regular consultation, and fellowships.

In terms of evaluation strategy, Bland, Dalgaard, Moo-Dodge, & Froberg (1985) found that gathering "satisfaction" data through participant surveys was the most often used strategy. Few external evaluation strategies were in evidence.

Site Visits
The five federally funded sites we visited reflected a variety of program models and strategies, both short-term and long-term. Michigan State University has a 3-month, on-/off-site fellowship that draws both community and university faculty in both tenure-track and non-

tenure-track positions. The Faculty Development Center in Waco, Texas serves all types of faculty (preceptors to tenure-track) via five separate programs that range in length from 1-day workshops to 3-month on-site fellowships.

A unique program was found at the University of Miami. The National Faculty Development Center runs a computer/telephone electronic network, publishes a monthly newsletter, and conducts regional and local workshops for affiliated sites. A year long fellowship for young family medicine faculty was found at the University of North Carolina at Chapel Hill. One or two fellows remain on-site throughout the year; most, however, enroll in a part-time (on-/off-site) version. Other programs for mid-career and senior faculty have also been created. At Duke University, the faculty development program runs two interrelated programs: a 1-year teaching fellowship and a seminar series. Fellows attend and even team-teach some of the seminars, which are attended by a variety of participants.

All five sites addressed teaching and to a lesser extent administration in their curricula. Three sites addressed research as well; two of these latter programs also included written communication. At least one nontraditional topic (i.e., ethics, survival skills) appeared in each program we visited.

Most programs evaluated their curricula, participants, and teachers quite extensively. Many critical insights into faculty development were identified by respondents at these sites; their comments and recommendations are incorporated into Chapter 10, "Guidelines for Implementing Faculty Development Programs."

References

Bland, C. J., Dalgaard, K., Moo-Dodge, M., & Froberg, D. A. (1985). Study of federally funded faculty development in family medicine from 1978–1981. *Family Medicine, 18*(2), 50–56.

Bland, C. J., Hitchcock, M., Anderson, W., & Stritter, F. T. (1986, March). *Study of graduates of family medicine faculty development fellowship programs.* Final report of the STFM Task Force on Faculty Development. Supported by the Robert Wood Johnson Foundation and HHS Contract #84 592 (p). Minneapolis: University of Minnesota.

Bland, C. J., Hitchcock, M. A., Anderson, W. A., & Stritter, F. T. (1987, August). Faculty development fellowship programs in family medicine. *Journal of Medical Education, 62*(8), 632–641.

Bland, C. J., Stritter, F. T. (1986a, December). *Final report on federal funding.* Deliverable #51, HRSA Contract #240-84-0077. Minneapolis: University of Minnesota.

Bland, C. J., Stritter, F. T., Schmitz, C., Aluise, J., & Henry, R. C. (1986b, December). *Final report on a model curriculum to prepare family medicine physicians to assume the role of new faculty members in either university- or community-based educational programs.* HRSA Contract #240-84-0077. Document #HRP0907077. Springfield, VA: National Technical Information Service.

Bland, C. J., & Stritter, F. T. (1988, July/August). Characteristics of effective family medicine faculty development programs. *Family Medicine, 20*(4), 282–288.

Gagne, R. M., & Briggs, L. I. (1974). *Principles of instructional design.* New York: Holt, Rinehart & Winston.

Gall, M. D. (1984). *Handbook for evaluating and selecting curriculum materials.* Boston: Allyn & Bacon.

Hitchcock, M. A., Anderson, W. A., Stritter, F. T., & Bland, C. J. (1988, January–February). Profiles of family practice faculty development fellowship graduates, 1978–1986. *Family Medicine, 20*(1), 33–38.

Payne, A. (1969). *The study of curriculum plans.* Washington, DC: National Education Association for the Study of Instruction.

Schmitz, C. C., Bland, C. J., & Stritter, F. T. (1986, March). *Survey of department heads and residency directors on selected faculty types and subsequent faculty development goals.* In-house report for HRSA Contract #240-84-0077. Minneapolis: University of Minnesota, Department of Family Practice and Community Health.

Stritter, F. T., Bland, C. J., & Youngblood, P. (1986, March). *Survey of exemplary medical faculty identified by 50 offices of medical education.* In-house report for HRSA Contract #240-84-0077. Chapel Hill: The University of North Carolina, Office of Research of Development for Education in the Health Professions.

Taba, H. (1962). *Curriculum development: Theory and practice.* New York: Harcourt, Brace & World.

Tyler, R. W. (1950). *Basic principles of curriculum and instruction.* Chicago: University of Chicago.

Index

Index